KUNDALINI AWAKENING AND MEDITATION

THE COMPLETE KUNDALINI GUIDE TO LEARN HIGHER MINDFULNESS, HEAL BODY, ANXIETY, SHAME. GAIN SPIRITUAL ENLIGHTENMENT WITH MEDITATION AND YOGA. RISES EMPATH, MIND POWER

Mindfulness Experience

DISCLAIMER

Copyright © Material 2020 all rights reserved.

TABLE OF CONTENTS
KUNDALINI AWAKENING

TABLE OF CONTENTS
KUNDALINI MEDITATION

KUNDALINI AWAKENING

THE COMPLETE KUNDALINI AWAKENING GUIDE TO ACHIEVE A HIGHER MINDFULNESS, HEAL YOUR BODY AND GAIN ENLIGHTENMENT WITH SPIRITUAL TRANSCENDENCE USING MEDITATION. INCREASE PSYCHIC INTUITION AND MIND POWER

Introduction

There is a buzz about Kundalini practices everywhere from spiritual circles to meditation/yoga classes. People are intrigued by what it is and how it can be used to create spiritual enlightenment, attain inner-peace, and increase physiological healing. This book will help you master various Kundalini awakening meditation techniques to facilitate your physical, mental, and spiritual well-being.

Kundalini awakening is just the beginning of awareness on so many levels: awareness of your own power, joy, psychic abilities, spiritual expansiveness, infinite potential and enlightenment with the source of all divine energy; the collective consciousness and awareness of all people and all beings and our collective ability to achieve transcendence; and overall high frequency vibration of light, love, and enlightenment.

The importance of our universe and the effect that we have on it will also be discussed to help improve our general outlook in our daily lives. The influence of karma and what goes around, comes around will be considered further to help reprogram our minds to a more positive outlook.

Chapter 1 The basics and understanding of kundalini Awakening

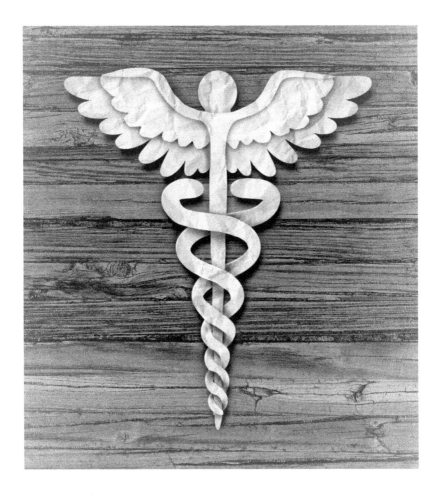

Some of us may be wondering: "What is Kundalini and how can it help us achieve inner peace?" Kundalini refers to the spiritual energy located within the spine. This energy takes the form of a female snake that is set coiled three times around the base of the spine. An utterly coiled form is how Kundalini first starts off for everyone. A Kundalini awakening is when this "snake" is slowly awoken and guided to slither up the channels of the spine until it finally reaches the twelfth chakra, activating each spiritual channel in the process.

This form of spiritual awakening is said to be one of the most life-changing. People often report living much lighter lives with balanced emotions and mind. It is possible that we have already achieved a Kundalini awakening without even realizing it, as these awakenings can happen from almost anything ranging from simple breathing exercises to a near-death experience.

As is the same with every practice, Kundalini awakening can take time. Yoga is one of the most common practices used in the awakening of Kundalini because it focuses mainly on opening up the channels of the spine.

Our Kundalini is made up of powerful vibrational energies that can be influenced and encouraged to strengthen and grow so that we may reach our higher spiritual awakening. Being able to understand the energies in our universe and the effect they have on all living creatures will help significantly in our understanding of the Divine mother within, our Kundalini.

Some gurus have dedicated their entire lives to the awakening and teaching of our Kundalini and the exercises that activate our spiritual growth. Because of them, we now have hundreds if not thousands of exercises available that will guide the awakening of our Kundalini and the improvement of our mental, physical, and spiritual health.

We may be wondering how on earth these kinds of awakenings could help us in our life or the lives of others. In the next chapter, we will discuss more all of the benefits of Kundalini and go more in depth about all the positive changes it will bring. Hopefully, this book will help provide the right guidance to those of us who want to achieve a higher level of mindfulness and inner peace.

How Kundalini Can Help

The practice of Kundalini awakening is used to help with almost every type of ailment. No matter what the cause, spiritual energy can always help in some way, even if it is bringing back hope to a life that has lost it all.

Through spiritual meditation we allow ourselves to open our mind's eye and see that which was first invisible to us. Meditation gives us the ability to see not only the potential in others but also the spiritual potential that we have within ourselves.

Allow our life energy to guide us through our journey, as Kundalini will not let us down. Once we become entirely in tune and with our Kundalini, life will start to fall into place. We are continually putting energies out into the world and attracting things back to us. Not all the time are the things that come back right, but we can learn to control that. What we give is what we get; that is the Kundalini way. Draw things to us using our new awakening and use them to our advantage.

A Kundalini awakening can have some physical effects on the body, including tremors, laughing, crying, and even a surge of energy. As Kundalini travels through the Nadi, it is widespread to have side effects related to the chakra that Kundalini is trying to travel through.

These may come to us as feelings of some emotional trial. For example, the root chakra focuses on security with one's self. We may feel vulnerable or invaluable while we try to break this blockage since it is those very feelings that are creating the block in the first place. Kundalini will guide us through these challenges and help us break the gates that are restricting the flow of the Nadi.

It is essential to understand what exactly a Kundalini awakening entails. Anyone and everyone can reach his or her awakening, but it does take time and practice. Even with this in mind, it is imperative not to get caught up in the same practice after achieving one successful experience. We may try to replicate this practice or specific meditation session to recreate the experience, which will most likely lead to a halt in improvement as our imaginations might start interrupting and replacing our healing.

Twelve chakras radiate through our Nadi. Each one usually has its own specific issue that blocks Kundalini's passage. Again, each experience will be different for each person, since everyone has his or her universal traumas and trials that he or she must face. Once we successfully break these walls, we can achieve a much better state of being, both physical and mental.

The first chakra is our root chakra; it is red and located in the region of the hips. This chakra has an in-body connection with the adrenals and is mainly attributed to our mental patience. Physical harm most commonly causes this blockage. These traumas could have been induced by childhood trauma or even a scare from a horrible car accident. Many forms of PTSD that leave scars in our soul will create the dam thus ceasing energy flow. The Sanskrit name for this chakra is Muladhara. It is also the base where Kundalini will begin to uncoil.

Our second chakra is orange and is located in the abdominal area. This energy is mainly linked to our sexual energies of the ovaries and testicles.

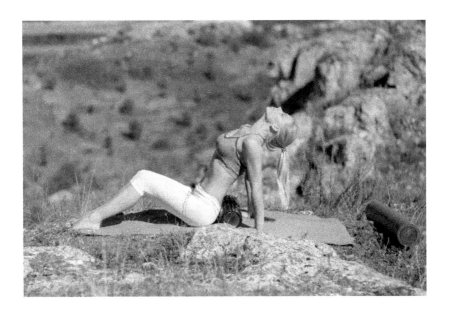

The block on this second level is usually emotional, and the spiritual gain of our awakening here is purity. If we let Kundalini guide us, she will lead us down the path of healing, so that our emotional scars may begin to fade. The Sanskrit name for our second chakra is Svadhishthana.

Third in line is the chakra located in our solar plexus, a bright yellow, known in Sanskrit as Manipura. The physical attributes of this blockage are usually within the pancreas and the main cause of this is our mentality. The gift Kundalini gives us from this awakening will be radiance. This might be a very difficult stage for some to overcome, but with the proper Kundalini Yoga exercises, the blockage can be cleared.

Fourth is our green chakra. This energy is located in the heart and will have physical connections in regard to this area. Relationships cause the issues that usually cause harm to our hearts. This doesn't only mean romance, but family and friend relationships as well. Our fourth chakra acts as our center, a balancing center for our energies. Results of clearing this chakra can bring about a shift in the sense of "me to we."

The fifth chakra in Sanskrit is known as Vishuddha and radiates a deep blue. This chakra resides in the throat and correlates to issues regarding communication. Words left unsaid will poison us from within our physical being. It is essential to keep a healthy state of communication, but this also can take some practice to completely perfect. Chatting a person's ear off for an hour is a lot different than sitting down and making sure we connect and get our statement across. Some of us may be waiting for somebody to apologize or vice versa, but the opportunity is only being delayed either for lack of or a misunderstanding in communication. Physical attributes for the fifth chakra will usually reside within the thyroid for this specific blockage. Once cleared, Kundalini will grant us the gift of unity.

Sixth is our purple chakra, located at the brow. The Sanskrit name for this chakra is Ajna, and the physical attribute for this energy is in the pituitary gland. Our vision is what creates the block for Kundalini's passage on this level. Once we can break through this blinding wall, the most common achievement is command within our lives.

Our seventh awakening resides in the white chakra of the crown; named Sahasrara in Sanskrit. This connection is with our pineal gland and is usually blocked by problems in our spirituality. When we achieve this awakening, the most common result is a higher form of consciousness.

The eighth chakra is a deep black and radiates above the head. This energy ties physical to our thymus gland and represents our power to move forward and begin a flow of change. Reaching an awakening on this level can grant one a type of shamanic awakening, allowing them to project onto different astral planes and travel in their dreams. Blockages in this chakra are usually themed by karma and even the loss of loved ones.

Ninth is our golden chakra, which is located about an arm's length above the head. Physical attributes for this energy are usually tied to the diaphragm. In a way, awakening this level will unlock a form of higher empathy. We should be able to pick up on the genes of other's souls. This ability will also help us achieve harmony by opening our soul and giving back to the earth.

The tenth chakra is brown and is rooted about a foot and a half underneath the ground. This energy is what grounds us and provides a sense of practicality. This chakra is linked to our bones and is linked to giving us a better sense of grounding and our ancestry to the earth. Having the ability to ground oneself is extremely important, especially while trying to meditate or recover from a stressful experience.

The eleventh chakra is a rose hue and surrounds our body, hands, and feet. Kundalini can help us shift supernatural and natural forces after this awakening, and may even give us a sense of leadership and ability. This chakra will link physically to the connective tissue.

Finally, our twelfth and final chakra is surrounding our entire auric field. This chakra has no color at all but is instead a bright energy. This energy connects to thirty-two in-body connections. This blockage will always be unique to each their own. Our twelfth aura represents our own personal, and spiritual path and the gift of this Kundalini awakening will be tailored to each person.

Once we master our Kundalini awakening, we are changing our entire outlook on the world. This shift should help uplift our soul and bring peace of mind and body.

Those of us that suffer from depression, anxiety, or posttraumatic stress disorder may find it a bit more difficult to clear the blockages that stand in Kundalini's way. A lot of these traumas will cause us to "lock" these gates so that our energies become stunted. It will take a lot more practice, but clearing those blocks can and will save our lives. The mind can be a dangerous thing when we do not know how to use it, but Kundalini can help make sure that no harm will come to us if we know how to ask for her help.

The Power and Benefits of Kundalini
Your nervous system response
Practicing Kundalini Yoga strengthens the body's nervous systems. Whenever you experience your body shaking when you do a downward dog pose or a plank pose, this is your nervous system reacting to these poses. The stronger your nerves become, the more you will be able to act in a

calm, collected and cool manner when faced with any kind of situation.

Willpower

We all want stronger willpower. With kundalini yoga, you get to empower and awaken your willpower at the center of your solar plexus or the third chakra, located at your navel point. When this happens, one of the things you may experience is a strong heat around this region, and this ultimately leads to better digestion and not just in terms of food but also your memories, good and bad as well as with self-doubt.

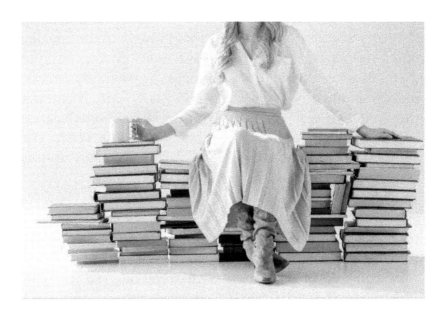

We are much more able to process and digest events that take place, and we are more focused on taking the necessary action to eradicate elements that cause us harm and this could be a person, a thing or even a situation.

Brain Power

Better brain power enables us to focus better. Practicing Kundalini enables us to get rid of the fogginess of our minds. With just a few minutes of rapid breathing, our minds become untangled of the cobweb of thoughts, we develop a crystal-clear mind, we are more alert and focused, and our concentration becomes better.

Our minds are less clouded with thoughts, and we have a better capacity to make sound decisions.

Creativity

Kundalini yoga brings out our inner creativity by releasing our stresses and worries. With this gone or reduced, our minds are better equipped to focus on the infinite possibilities of an issue or solving a problem. When we practice Kundalini yoga, we alternate our breathing through the nostrils-this brings our mind and body balance to both the right and left hemispheres of the brain. We stimulate and use both sides of the brain to act, analyze, feel, visualize and imagine.

Embracing

Kundalini also opens up our fourth chakra, the heart center. Doing the tree post enables us to root our chakra with security, and this makes us feel stronger and steadier like a strong, rooted tree that is planted firmly on Earth. We also become more open and trusting with the higher power, trusting that we will be provided with what we need when the time is right.

We do not feel like our life has ended when we do not get the job we want, we do not feel like there is nothing to live for when the person we love has left us, we do not feel depressed when we fail an exam. Whatever that happens, we go through these situations with an attitude of acceptance.

Compassionate communication

Poses like the Shoulder Stand opens our throat center or the fifth chakra in Kundalini yoga. This makes us more forgiving and compassionate, and it makes us less judgmental. We are always reminded to give gratitude and to address the people we speak to and come into contact. Whenever there is an issue that is bothering you, you find the best way and positive way to express yourself in a way that everyone understands and without confrontation.

Awakened intuition

Whenever we are faced with an issue or a problem, we spend so much time thinking about the pros and cons when in fact, we already have an answer to that problem. Deep inside us, we already know what we want to do, or we often have a gut feeling of what would happen or could happen. Kundalini yoga enables us to exercise the ability to pause and listen to this gut feeling of ours. It helps us quieten our mind so that our thoughts become still and we can hear what our heart yearns for. This will ultimately make us better in dealing and solving problems.

Making wise choices

Practicing yoga brings out the best in you. Any form of yoga you choose to do, you will end up eliminating bad behaviors from your system from removing yourself voluntarily from toxic situations, ending your contact with toxic people, stopping negative habits such as drinking, smoking and doing drugs. You will become better and start consuming healthier foods, doing things to protect animals and the environment, serving others in charitable causes and giving back to the community. In other words, you do things consciously to bring out the best in you.

Kundalini also helps bring a strong connection between our soul as well as our purpose here on earth. This is where we start making great strides towards living as enlightened people. So, in practicing Kundalini yoga, practice it for yourself. It will add depth and richness to your life.

Chapter 2 What Kundalini awakening is and what the best and the easiest way to achieve it is

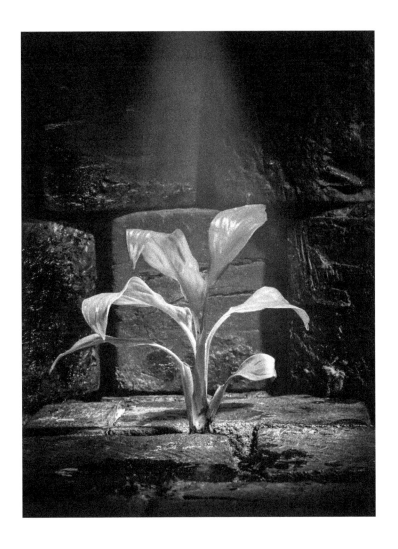

The kundalini energy is as mysterious as it is powerful. When you begin to work with it, you will realize why it is a practice that many people spend their whole lives performing. To work with this energy is to seek the divine, to reveal the true nature of reality and find our innermost potential as humans. These are no small achievements. They require dedication and hard work to accomplish. Overall the kundalini is consciousness manifest inside each human, to access and work with this energy to dance with Shiva and Shakti, unfolding your own personal universe.

When we reference kundalini awakening, we are really talking about the acknowledgment of this energy. In essence to awaken this energy is to work with it intentionally and live with it, rather than separate from it. When we begin to work with this energy, we awaken it, it may still be coiled, but it is no longer dormant. As the serpent uncoils, we find it shakes off its slumber and begins to move through the nadis and chakras. This awakening is only the beginning of a powerful and esoteric transformation. When we awaken kundalini, we awaken ourselves and take the first steps on a holy path to wholeness.

We have seen the relationship between kundalini, nadis, and chakras. As a preliminary practice to kundalini work, we need to familiarize ourselves with the chakras and their attributes. Working with these energy centers helps to not only move the flow of energy but also to help analyze any personal issues we have with our physical self. Meditating on the chakras is a great way to self-examine, almost like a self-psychoanalysis. We can learn about what factors in our physical lives are causing us pain or preventing us from progressing through life. We can learn to live with our subtle energetic body in mind at all times, learning to think with these concepts and make them a core part of our human experience.

This introduction of energetic concepts into our daily lives is the first step to developing a practice that will act to wake the kundalini energy. We need to approach these ideas cautiously, with patience and respect. These practices are transformative in nature, they will change your life, and we want to ensure that our lives change for the better.

We have learned that kundalini is a fragment of the source of the universe. By learning to live with this notion on a day to day basis, we can familiarize ourselves with this energy, letting it become a part of our everyday life and thus rebuilding a relationship that is mostly lost in western society. These small steps to building this relationship are just as important as the practices themselves. We need to acknowledge kundalini's role in our lives, respect that role, and then actively work with it to empower ourselves.

Many spiritual communities hold strict guidelines and rules as to how to practice working with kundalini. This is fool-hearted. There is no one way to start these practices, and not one way that will work for everyone. There are general paths to take when approaching this energy, but overall anyone can define their own path as they start on this journey. The practices are all-inclusive and universal as means to dance with the divine. It is every human's birthright to experience these gifts from the universe.

Prepping Our Energetic Bodies

When we begin to develop a practice to awaken our kundalini energy, we need to consider our routine as it is. Have you ever practiced yoga or meditation? What spiritual world view do you adhere to? Your weekly routine with work, family, and hobbies will all be affected by your new practice, so we need to find time to organize and practice these arts. We must also talk about the repercussions of prematurely sparking a kundalini awakening. This can do irreversible damage to your brain and body.

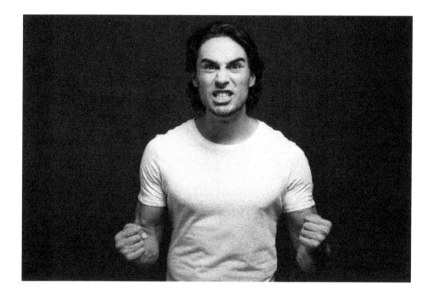

Many people try to perform advanced exercises that they are not prepared for, resulting in an energetic upheaval that their minds are not ready for. This premature awakening can come in many forms. Some people who don't even practice these exercises can experience these awakenings. This is common with the use of psychedelic drugs, or other lifestyles that stimulate the kundalini energy. Some people can be leading perfectly healthy lives and awaken their kundalini.

This is troublesome because the individuals do not realize what is happening, and it stresses them out, leading to unneeded doctor's visits or mental disturbance.

It is highly recommended that we start a simple meditation practice to prepare our minds and bodies for the kundalini practices. Working with visualization and chakra energy work are the best starting points with your meditation practice. When we work with these energies, we need to learn how to feel and recognize the effects that are taking place. Familiarizing ourselves with the movement of energies in and around our bodies is key to recognizing that our practices are working. These energies are subtle, so we need to develop our awareness and be mindful of our energetic bodies.

We can learn to develop this mindfulness by taking time each day to consider our energy. What does our overall energy feel like today? Or what is the energy of the office this day? These simple contemplative exercises will help us learn to live with our energetic bodies rather than separate from them. This may seem very simple, but you will soon learn that noticing the energetic makeup of a room is tough when there's so much going on. Learning to feel this energy is the first step to being able to manipulate and move it.

There are many ways to go about casual energy work on a daily basis. One of the most common ways is to utilize breath. The next time you are stressed or upset, make it a point to feel the tense energy. Really feel its tension and discomfort. Now take a deep breath and see how you feel.

Do this breath ten times and see how your energy changes. It will typically be more comfortable and easier to manage. This simple breathing exercise is the starting point of your new path to kundalini awakening. It literally starts with one deep breath.

Let's take time to explore more techniques and methods that can be used to align our minds with the energetic currents all around us. These techniques are not mandatory but are the proven most effective ways to reach our goals with the kundalini energy. Yoga and meditation will be our main focus for the preliminary exercises. These practices are rooted in Indian culture, just like the concepts of kundalini. We can start a simple practice performing these arts to help us ease into the lifestyle that is centered on awakening the kundalini energy.

As we see in the modern West, these practices are often used for physical benefits only, even though there is an invaluable amount of spiritual wealth to be found with these arts. For our intents and purposes in this book, we will focus on these practices to prepare our minds and bodies for our more advanced kundalini work. These practices can be practiced with what we have learned about chakras as well. With this in mind, we will develop a routine practice that we can practice as much as possible to prepare for our awakening. This includes including chakra energy work into our practices.

When we work with kundalini, we can take common practices like meditation and yoga, then include a kundalini-centric mindset to filter the practices through. While practicing meditation and yoga will stimulate your energetic body, we need to approach kundalini directly through these ancient practices to truly awaken the serpent.

29

The following practices are great for beginners to start working with their energetic systems. Let's explore these practices as we begin.

Meditation

The practice of meditation aims to clear the mind of chaotic thoughts and memories. This state of no-thought is the preferred mindset to be in when we are working with our energy.

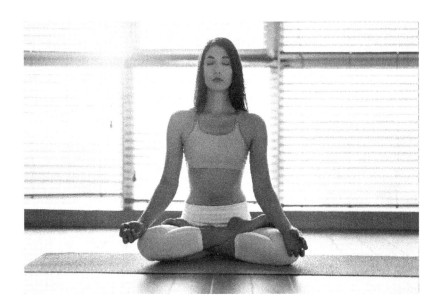

With a clear mind, we can better acknowledge our energy at work. We will not be distracted by the constant onslaught of the chaotic mind.

Meditation has found popularity in the West, but mainly for physical benefits. The calming of the mind and peaceful nature of this practice is beneficial, but we need to focus heavily on our energetic bodies to achieve our desired results of awakening the kundalini energy.

The practice is difficult to define with only one definition. There are so many varying techniques and traditions that a simple definition just won't suffice. The rise in popularity of meditation in the West accompanied yoga and concepts of kundalini in the 1960s. As it found its way to the West, it adopted many different techniques and practices to build a complex and powerful art form that it has become today.

A standard definition of meditation can be any practice whose ultimate goal is to clear the mind of thought and offer a sense of expanded consciousness for the practitioner. These practices can include; breath work, visualization, musical trance, mantra, and a variety of other techniques that promote these ideas. Overall this practice is another universal exercise that adheres to no spiritual or religious affiliation, but rather offers a beneficial experience to anyone who's willing to dedicate some time to the practices. These techniques have been used by humans for thousands of years to access hidden knowledge and balance the chaotic mind.

To achieve the calm state of mind that meditation offers is invaluable, there are no other practices that claim to achieve these outcomes. To achieve this, one-pointed stillness is one of the main goals of meditation. In all major religions and spiritual traditions, this stillness is key to open the body and mind to the unseen natural forces at work all around us and within us. If we are distracted by our own thoughts, we may miss important insights or realizations that are much needed to achieve our desired goals. This is where the concept of the present moment comes into play a well. Many of the thoughts that are so distracting during meditation stem from being stuck in the past or future. By staying in the present moment, we can avoid these distracting thoughts.

Yoga

The word yoga is loosely translated as 'union' in English. This is a reference to the union of body and mind. This union is attainable with yogic practice, not unlike the union we seek to induce between Shakti and Shiva with the awakening of the kundalini energy.

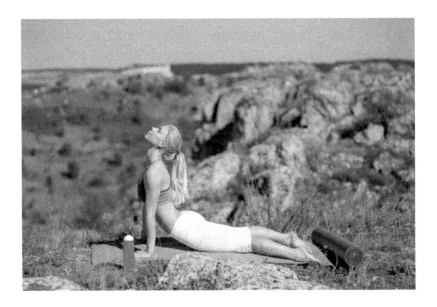

This yogic union is a great precursor to the union of kundalini. If we can properly experience the union of body and mind, seeing that we are not separate from the mind, then we can understand the principles of kundalini more fluently. Yoga lives hand in hand with meditation. Consider finding the union of body and mind, then sitting to contemplate or simply live in the experience. It is also thought that if your body is limber and flexible that you will be able to sit for longer periods of meditation without experiencing pain or tightened muscles. These two practices, paired together, are crucial as preliminary exercises to awaken kundalini.

Working with Chakras

The disc-like nature of the chakras allows us to feel their energy flowing through us. As a basic practice, we can sit down and try to feel this energy with our hands. Simply sitting with our chakras is the first step to building this relationship with our energetic bodies. From the chakras outward, we can feel our body's energy. Many people in the West know this as an aura, an energetic bubble that surrounds our physical body. This is the energy that gets agitated when you can feel someone else's energy, or when someone gets into your personal space uninvited.

As a preliminary practice to awakening, the kundalini energy is to learn to feel these chakras. You can begin by sitting comfortably and breathing deep. Try and visualize your chakras, their colors, and motions. Notice if you get any distinct feelings as you try to feel these energetic centers. You can even practice deep breathing techniques to help stimulate your chakras:

- Stay seated comfortably.
- Take ten deep breaths and clear your mind.
- On the eleventh breath exhale as much as you can.
- Visualize the root chakra, its color, or yantra.
- Exhale, noting any distinct feelings or movements.
- Repeat this exercise with all the chakras.

You may continue this exercise after the crown chakra, starting over with the root chakra again and working your way upwards. Visualize your aura as you continue this cycle. Are there any distinct changes or movements that take place?

If at first, you do not feel any significant movement do not be discouraged. It may take a few practice sessions for you to attune yourself to these energy centers. As you progress, you will become more mindful of the chakras, learning their movements and recognizing which of your personal chakras need the most attention at first.

Visualization

The practice of visualization is a crucial aspect of any spiritual practice. Visualization techniques go along with the idea that we need to be in control of our thoughts to truly be able to move the energy through our bodies. Visualization techniques aim to busy the mind, but not in the chaotic way that thoughts come and go normally. Being able to visualize certain images or scenarios allows us to be in control of our mind and its need to be constantly working.

Many visualization techniques are performed by imagining the mundane day to day tasks. For instance, visiting a friend or preparing a meal. These techniques work to help us control the images in our minds, thus controlling our thoughts. If we can create and manage intentional scenarios and images, we can better control our thoughts in day to day life as well as during our kundalini practices.

Practice Space

One way to organize our practices on our path to kundalini awakening is by creating a personal space to practice within. This space will act as the home of your practice. You will perform your routine in this space as often as possible. The area dedicated to your practice does not have to be a full room or elaborate chamber. This space can be a quaint corner of your bedroom or other small space that is yours.

Find a space that you not be disturbed in. Maintaining focus is crucial to a successful practice, and we don't want any distractions from pets, roommates, or children. When you have chosen your space, you need to thoroughly clean it and make sure it fits for your practice.

Once it is clean, you can decorate it as you wish. Really make it your own and have décor and items that you can be relaxed around. It is common to have a small table in this space where you can have incense, candles, music, or other items to help with your practice. Be sure your space is comfortable and that you have a nice cushion or pillow to sit upon.

When decorating this area, be sure to use images and items that are kundalini friendly.

Have a tapestry with the chakra's images and colors, or have serpent images and symbols. If you adhere to a certain religion, keep your deities and religious items in this space as well. This area will become an altar to your dedicated practice.

The use of a personal space helps us keep our practice consistent. If we do not have a place to practice, we are less likely to adhere to our routine, straying from the path. This space will also act to amplify the effectiveness of your energetic work.

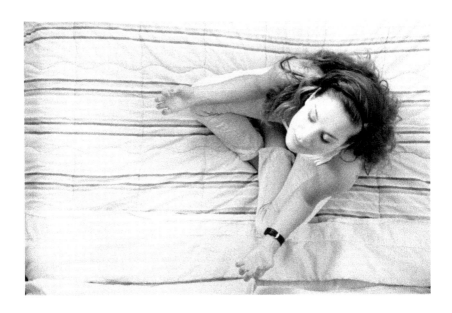

You will begin to notice that even glancing at the space will start to prepare your mind for your routine. This area will become spiritually potent the more you use it. It is as if your mind is aware that you are about to begin your routine and start without your intention!

Be sure to keep this area clean and comfortable. There will be candle wax, incense, and the collection of dust, but be sure to clean it once or twice a month. Without proper cleansing, this space could potentially gather energy and get blocked, as rooms tend to do. With a dedicated practice area ready to go, you will be on your way to having a daily practice in no time.

Chapter 3 What Prana is and how it works

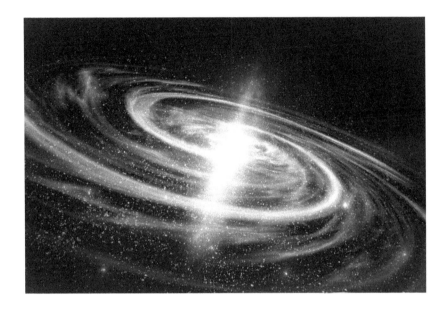

Prana is the all-pervading energy that exists inside you and all around you. It is called by many names and terms, yet they all refer to the same divine energy: prana. Even some people claim so far that since prana is everywhere and that it cannot be destroyed, then perhaps prana is God. There are conflicting schools of thought on this matter, but the majority believes that prana only comes from God, but it is not God. Still, the nature of prana remains the same: It is everywhere; it is infinite; it cannot be destroyed but is transmuted from one state into another; and that everything – both visible and invisible – is made of prana. Without prana, then there is no life. From this perspective, it is not hard to say that perhaps prana, indeed, is God. However, this is something that you may have to decide on your own,

How to control prana

This is a secret that you must learn to and understand. You will find this extremely helpful especially when you finally take the actual steps to awaken the Kundalini. When it comes to controlling prana, you should remember that prana follows thought. This means that you can control prana with your mind. But how do you do it? Well, the answer is actually simpler than you might think. It is through visualization. Yes, you just have to imagine it.

However, this is more than doing a simple imaginary act. You should engage as many senses as possible. For example, if you want to draw prana into your hand, then you can visualize prana, like a flowing river, flowing into your hand. Do not just see it in your mind's eye, but also try to feel it, even hear it and smell it. The more senses are involved the better it will be. There are, however, two important senses that you should ensure to focus on — the senses of sight (seeing) and feeling.

Again, remember that energy follows thought. To truly engage this energy, you should use visualization. Through visualization, you can effectively direct prana. There are, of course, other ways to control prana; but as far as working on your Kundalini is involved, then the best way to do it is with the use of visualization while you are engaged in meditation.

Do not think of this as a mere exercise with your imagination. You must also have faith that what you visualize is also real. Keep in mind that prana can take any form, color, and shape; and all it takes is for you to control it with your mind.

There is also what is known as tactile visualization. This is also effective. If you find it hard to visualize and "see" things in your mind's eye, then you may want to learn tactile visualization instead. Tactile visualization is where you rely solely on your feelings. For example, instead of visualizing the sight of a fire in your hand to produce heat, you can just visualize or imagine your hand getting warmer and warmer, even without having to "see" a fire in your hand. However, it should be noted that it is still best to get used to doing visualization using as many senses as possible. Do not worry if you think you cannot do it in your first few attempts. It may take some practice before you can get used to it, but it is definitely doable, and you can do it.

Here is a simple exercise to help you learn to control prana:

Focus on your hand. You can use either your left or right hand. Now, visualize the energy in your body. You can see it in any way you want. The most common way of visualizing energy is by seeing it as white light. Now, see and feel this energy flow and accumulate in your hand. Keep charging your hand. You can also direct and accumulate energy/prana in other parts of your body.

Energy is often felt as something warm. Hence, if you accumulate energy in your hand, you may be able to tell if you are able to do it correctly if you feel that your hand gets warmer.

Another sign of energy is when you feel a tingling sensation. This is often felt on the palm of your hand.

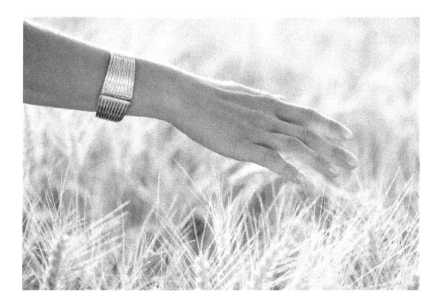

Take note that energy is inside you and all around you. The energy inside you is referred to as personal energy. There is also what is known as universal energy. This is the unlimited energy that exists all around you.

Understanding the nature of prana

Prana is said to be everywhere. It is inside you and all around you. No life can exist without prana. Prana is also in the breath. Hence, there is a famous practice known as pranayama, which is a practice of controlling one's prana by controlling the breath. Another nature of prana is that it cannot be killed or destroyed. Instead, it can only change or be transmuted from one state into another. It is interesting to note, that conventional science has also proven this teaching, that energy cannot be destroyed; it only changes.

Everything in the universe swims in an ocean of energy. Perhaps this is also how everything is said to be connected. Hence, the web of life.

Prana or energy can also be used for various purposes. It is not just for awakening the Kundalini. Many people use it for healing, such as in reiki and in pranic healing. It can also be used for many other purposes, even for evil. Indeed, prana is everything and everything is composed of prana. Although prana may be seen as one and the same, it should be noted that its quality might vary. When you use prana, only focus on harnessing positive energy.

There are many other ways to direct prana, although the simplest and usual way of doing it is by visualization. Other known ways include dancing, chanting, and certain movements, among others.

Prana is considered important to humans. People with low prana are often more prone to getting sick, while people with lots of prana are more likely to be active and healthy.

Prana or chi has been in existence for centuries; in fact, ancient writings also talked about prana. Mind you, these writings can be traced back to before the time of Christ. However, although prana has been known and used for so long, it is not yet accepted by conventional science. Still, this does not mean that it is not real. Just because science cannot explain something does not mean that it does not exist.

The Energy of Prana

This is even something modern scientists believe to be true. For years, people believed that everything was just a bunch of molecules and atoms.

However, when they took a deeper look at these structures, it was discovered that they were made up of energy. This means that without prana, nothing could live. That is why it is important that you know how to use and understand prana.

When you meditate, your system is charged with prana. Researchers have used Kirlian photography, a kind of photography that lets you see people's energy and aura, to prove this point. That is why meditation is so important. The crazy thing is that the power of personal energy is not new, yet people are just now learning about it.

The prana that lives within you is known as personal prana and the prana that lives in the world is known as universal prana. Both sources can be tapped into and used at any time. Most gurus will teach you that using personal prana is not efficient because it will drain you physically. Therefore, if you need to use quite a bit of energy, it is best to tap into the universal energy.

To help you better understand prana, we are going to look at how to control and use it. This will allow you to feel it.

Controlling Prana

The first thing you need to know before you start to control prana is that it follows thought. One of the most effective ways of controlling prana is to use your mind. How do you use your mind to do this? The secret is visualization. Visualization is often seen as the sense of sight. While this may be true, you can increase your visualization power by engaging all of your other senses. If you are trying to visualize a dog, you do not just see it, but you also feel, hear, and smell it. Feeling is a very important sense to use when you are working with prana. You want to feel the energy as it moves. In fact, you can easily control prana with only the sense of feel. This is known as tactile visualization.

Enough talking about it, let's actually look at how to control prana. This first exercise is only a visualization, but it will help you in getting used to working with prana.

Start by relaxing your hand and focusing on it.

Now, start to feel and see your personal prana flowing within you. Visualize as your prana gathers in your hand. Feel the accumulation of energy.

With practice, you will notice your energy pooling in that hand. Remember, try to use as many senses as you can.

This is going to be a lot easier than it may seem once you actually do it. While doing this practice, you have to stay focused on what you are trying to do. You may find thoughts of "my mind is playing tricks on me," creeping into your head. You have to push these out. That is your doubt talking. Make sure you practice this regularly, and you will eventually be able to control your prana.

Let's take a look at another basic exercise.

Rub your hands together until you can feel the warmth in your palms. Place your hands in front of you like you were holding a baseball. Picture yourself pulling Universal prana into that ball you have between your hands.

Prana is able to take on any form, so you can picture it any way that you want. For beginners, it is best to view it as a white light. Watch it and feel it as it moves and gathers into the space between your hands.

Can you feel it? Really focus your thoughts and mind on it and allow your visualization to take over. Allow yourself to be open to the sensations and relax and allow the universal energy to flow.

After you have learned how to use these basic prana exercises, you will start to notice how easy it is to manipulate and use prana. As you get more comfortable with this, you will be able to use prana in many different ways.

The Nature

The nature of prana is that it cannot ever be destroyed, but it can be altered. This is why everything is said to be eternal. Prana isn't limited by time and space. It knows no bounds and is endless. Many people view prana as God. People who can control it have the ability to harness great power. However, in order to successfully do this, you have to have a well-focused mind. This is yet another reason why meditation is so important because it will train you to use the power of your mind more effectively.

Prana is very sensitive. If you lose your focus, the prana will dissipate. In order to control prana, you have to control your mind. Don't stress about this, though, it will come with time.

Chapter 4 The Akasha

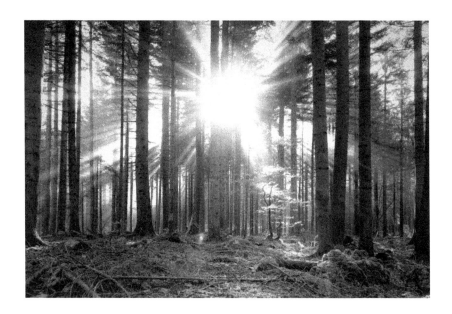

We will talk about the four main elements in the next chapter, but first, we are going to talk about Akasha or the source. It is believed to be the fifth element in which the four other elements originate from. It is the origin of all things. There are some people who view Akasha to be the god principle. While it is not technically an element, meaning you can't physically create it, it does possess all elements. It is most closely associated with the colors black and white. It does not conform to space or time. It is infinite. It is the beginning and the end. It's easy to see why many people associated Akasha with God. They are both described in similar manners, so it is perfectly fine to view Akasha as God if it helps.

Since Akasha possesses all of the qualities of the elements and holds all colors, mastering Akasha will give you the power to master the elements. This is by no means as simple as it may sound. To master this power requires a very high level of spiritual development and maturity. Still, it is something that can be done while you continue along your spiritual quest.

Just like the elements, everything in the Universe that can and cannot be seen comes from Akasha. Nothing is able to escape the power of Akasha because it is everywhere.

Some even believe that Akasha holds the records of everything that has happened or will ever happen of the past, present, and future. With a developed clairvoyant ability, a person can tap into the records of the Akasha and share somebody's future. This is the method that many psychics and diviners use.

Akasha lives within the astral plane. This is the reason for the spaceless and timeless ability of the astral plane. It is also important to know that every physical being has an astral counterpart. In fact, everything exists in the astral plane before they are given a physical body. Every plane is the same. They only differ in the types of vibrations that live within them. It is easy to understand that Akasha has the highest vibration of all the elements.

You do not have to master Akasha to benefit from its power. Mastery can end up taking years or your entire life to achieve, so it is important to start using its benefits now. When you start to work with Akasha, you will start to notice improvements in your psychic abilities, your chakras, and your energy overall.

There are some practitioners who do nothing but try to master the power of Akasha since it is the key to all things. However, gaining psychic powers and the like should not be your reasoning behind your spiritual focus. Gaining these powers is just a byproduct of awakening your Kundalini energy. You should focus on gaining spiritual maturity and not be blinded by gaining power.

Akasha is also sometimes referred to as intelligence. Whether or not this intelligence will help you or hinder you will determine your life; whether you become blessed or are someone who gets knocked around by life. Both types of people can easily be seen in life. There are some that seem to get everything they ever wanted and others who work their butt off but get nowhere. It is that person's ability, either unconsciously or consciously, to allow this power to influence their life.

A common practice that can be done to help Akasha work for you is to get up each morning before the sun rises and as the sun comes up, and before it passes at an angle of 30 degrees, look up to the sun and bow down to Akasha, thanking it for keeping you where you need to be. At another point during the day, anytime, look at the sky and bow again. Once the sun has set, look up at the sky and bow again. This is not being done to a god or anything. This is being done for the empty space that has held you in place. You will be amazed how your life will change when you do this.

Without Akasha, just like without prana or air, you cannot exist. It is easy to understand that without air you can't live. You need air to breathe. The vast majority of people do not even acknowledge the air around them, yet they are constantly using it. It can't be seen, but we know it's there.

48

That is how Akasha works. We cannot see it or touch it, but it is there and it is necessary for our survival.

In southern India, in the town of Karnataka, there is a temple dedicated to Annapoorneshwari. At the back of the temple, an inscription is written in Hale Kannada that describes how to design an airplane. It talks about how it should be constructed and it talks about how when the machine is flown, it will disrupt the ether. They believed that if the Akasha is disturbed, humans wouldn't be able to live peacefully. When Akasha is disturbed, psychological disturbances will become prevalent. This disruption has happened and we must live with it, but we can still use Akasha and actively work to improve ourselves with its power.

Accessing the Akashic Records

A person can access their own Akashic records without a lot of training or practice because they are their own. This is very different from accessing somebody else's, which takes a lot more practice and spiritual maturity. They can be accessed from anywhere and at any time.

There are some directions that you should make sure you follow. When you do decide to connect with your own records, what is best for you will show itself. You do not have to have advanced psychic abilities to access your own records. All you need to be is alive and have a true heartfelt desire to get started. Lastly, you have to believe in yourself.

Accessing the Akashic records is not something that only a few people are allowed to do, and as long as you have a pure heart, it will not be that difficult. Anybody can do it in many different ways. What plays the biggest part in this is the motivation behind it.

I am going to provide you with a quick practice to access your own records. Accessing your own is easier because you carry yours with you, so to speak.

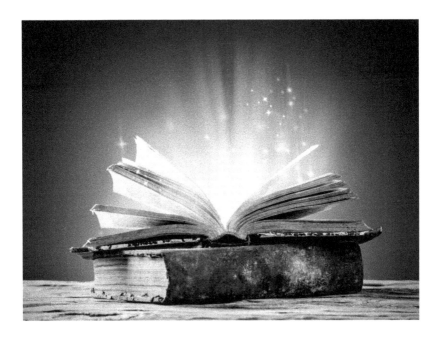

This means you do not have to access the hall of records that live within the astral plane. While it may not be difficult to access your own records, there are a few prerequisites. The first is being able to get into a meditative state. You have to know how to place your current thoughts to the side and be open to the information that you may receive.

Secondly, you must be willing to accept and reveal whatever is in your records. You can receive disturbing information from past lives and the like, so you have to make sure you are in a place where those things can be accepted. If you tend to avoid problems or steer clear of challenges in your daily life, how are you going to face this type of information in your records?

It is also a good idea to have a compassionate understanding of humanity so that your reading is meaningful. For example, you could learn that you were a slave owner in a past life. For most, this will be seen as a horrible thing, but that thought will close your heart and cause the reading to stop. Just because you were a slave owner doesn't mean you were a cruel person. You could have treated them fairly and kindly, but it was the norm for those times and you had very few options available to you.

Having not moved past this past life could be what is affecting your current life. That is why it's important that you go into your readings understanding that past lives happen the way they do because of those times. The more understanding you have of life, the better your readings will be.

It is very important that you have a reason for doing this and not just "let's see what I get" kind of attitude. You could end up receiving a lot of information that may not be influential to your current life. You want to be as clear and direct as possible.

To start, ask something along the lines of, "This (briefly describe your problem) is what I have been trying to work on, and I think there is more to it than what I know presently. If this is true, please send me information on how and when this problem started."

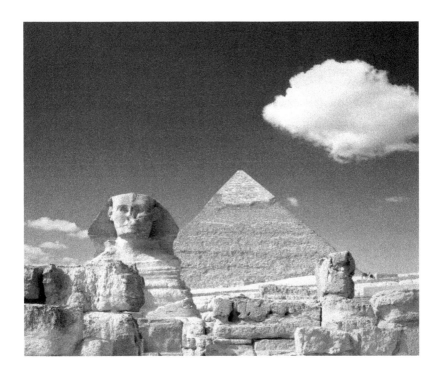

The way you get your answer will depend on your psychic strength. You could receive something from the past history to present, as a video clip or picture on your vision screen. You could hear a clip of music that means something. You could taste, smell, or feel something. Or, you could just realize that you know something. It could also be a combination. Allow this information to come in and then ask a few clarifying questions if you need to. Once you are done, close the session with gratitude. You were given what you need to know in that moment.

You will want to have a journal and write down the things you learn immediately so that you don't forget anything. As far as knowing if it is accurate, you will just know. It will make sense to you. Sometimes people will experience changes, have pains disappear, and some experience a cold before they become better. These don't happen all the time or to everybody.

There may be times when the reading does not resonate with you, but it is still accurate. This is when you have received a reading has revealed an uncomfortable truth. Do not allow yourself to fall into denial. These readings can lead to big changes.

When you first do this, keep your readings brief. There is a lot of information in your records, so you must keep yourself focused. You do not want to end up overwhelmed. This can cause inaccuracy.

I also must caution you this, once you get used to access your own records, you could be tempted to access other peoples'. You should not do this EVER unless you have their explicit consent. Reading another person's records without their consent is like breaking into their house and stealing personal information. No matter how benevolent your reasoning may be, it is still wrong. Now, you can read family members' records without consent to the extent of what is relevant to you.

The most important thing is to make sure that you treat these records with respect because Akasha knows everything.

Chapter 5 Auras and how to see them

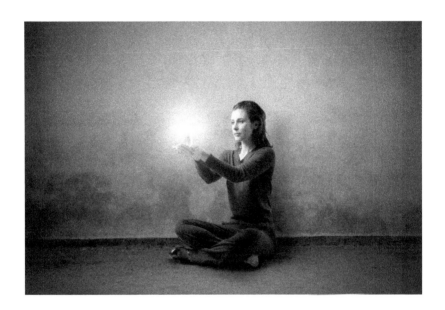

What exactly is an aura? You have surely heard the term before, but it may not be clear what it is exactly. Basically, every single person has one. In fact, all living beings do, but we are going to focus on us, humans. It's the energy field around people that gives you a feel for who they are as a person. Auras can be seen as colorful light emanating from somebody or energy sensed from somebody without touching them that can tell you information about the individual's personality. Reading auras can be tricky and requires practice to master it.

Auras have been recognized worldwide and throughout history as three-dimensional, oval, egg-shaped fields of electromagnetic energy that surround all living and nonliving things. Mystics and other clairvoyants have long described this phenomenon, often describing them as waves and bands of colors radiating out from the subject of observation. Halos depicted in religious iconography are another way of portraying this curiosity.

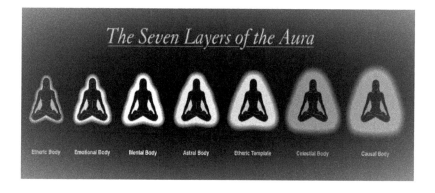

The aura contains emotional, physical, cognitive, and spiritual information about the person, and is essentially a reflection of the person's energetic composition. This includes their current life as well as past ones. The size and colors of the aura continuously fluctuate depending on the current state and health of the being, and can change significantly over time.

People with a lot of charisma have stronger fields, and have an ability to influence people with their power. People who are confident and healthy have more resilient auras, and are better at deflecting energy coming their way.

Those who are unsure of themselves and suffer from emotional and physical problems will have thinner auras, and struggle to defend themselves from external influences.

In spite of these difference, the aura of an ordinary person, even healthy ones, is not very stable, and reflects the ever-changing moods and compulsive thinking common to humans.

It is only with great spiritual work that the aura becomes steady and unwavering — a reflection of the training of the mind. With greater awareness comes an understanding of the value of the aura, and the need to proactively protect oneself against negativity, the same way we protect ourselves against illness and weather conditions.

An aura can expand or shrink according to the type of interaction. In general, expanding auras indicate a more expansive, happier state of wellbeing, while retracting energy is a sign of shrinking back into oneself.

A healthy aura will experience changes, but will have a more durable nature and be able to stay balanced in the midst of environmental difficulties. The aura changes based upon numerous conditions, including health, weather, and other environmental stimuli, interpersonal interactions, thought patterns, emotions, and spiritual practice.

Another important factor is the movement of the planets. The position of the heavenly bodies affects all in subtle and sometimes not so subtle ways. The aura actually contains the individual's astrological blueprints, and different signs tend to have unique characteristics in their auras that reflect their underlying tendencies.

Most auras are relatively calm with bursts of activity, and are quite small in comparison to their potential. In general, positive auras attract and negative auras repel. An important exception to this rule is when manipulative people use deceit to appear attractive, when underneath they are operating from low motivations.

They are able to wear a kind of energetic mask that fool others into believing them, unless they are attuned to a deeper level of insight. Other situations include feeling overwhelmed by a bright aura because it opens you up beyond your comfort zone, or being threatened by one because it reminds you of your own shortcomings.

Auras are extensions of individual souls, but it is possible for two or more auras to merge momentarily, temporarily, or for longer periods of time in a phenomenon called "auric coupling". Perhaps two friends had an in-depth conversation, or two people were recently physically intimate.

A person's aura can show up as a color or multiple colors surrounding a person's body. To practice seeing someone's aura, you could ask a friend if they could stand in front of a white background. It does not have to be their whole body, just head and shoulders are fine if you don't have a large enough background. This is the best way for a beginner to practice as the neutral background will make any colors that appear around them pop out clearly. Other colors can be distracting and cause bias, so ask them to wear the most neutral clothing possible. Try not to be in an environment you think will distract you or cause you to lose focus.

As well as seeing someone's aura, it is also possible to sense someone's aura energetically. This is slightly easier than seeing the aura, and you've likely sensed someone's aura in the past unwittingly. You can first practice sensing auras with yourself, and your own energetic presence. It is easy, and there are two ways of doing this. The first way is to rub your palms together to stimulate them, and then hold them apart from each other. Slowly begin bringing them closer together, noticing the energy you feel, the changes, the increase in energy as you bring them closer together. The other way is similar. Press your palms together with some strength for 30 seconds to a minute. Then pull them apart, and slowly bring them back into each other, the same as in the first method. In both methods, notice how you could sense the energy of your palms the closer they got, even though they were not touching at all?

Aura reading both visually and energetically is a useful skill for the psychic because it helps you get a sense of the person you are doing a reading for – what they are like as a person and what their current emotional and mental state is. You can pick up on any worries or reservations they may have, as well as what mood they're in coming into the reading.

Having this knowledge can help you tailor the reading to the subject. As a psychic, you will find that no two people, and therefore no two readings, will be the same. You may want to use different techniques, tools, and ways of explaining premonitions to someone based on the insights you have picked up from them.

Your aura is your energy field. It is a reflection of yourself and your current state of being. It can be weighed down and get clogged with negative energies, so here's how to cleanse and refresh it.

Your aura may also be stagnant because you are in a stagnant spot in your life. Do some deep digging and introspection to see if you can get to the bottom of this. Is there some aspect of your life that you do not like? Do you feel unfulfilled? Is it time for a change? No amount of deep breathing is going to answer these questions. If you think they are applicable to how you feel, you are going to have to tackle them, no matter how hard it may be. For your own wellbeing, you need to get to the bottom of what aspect of your life needs an adjustment.

If you remain stuck energetically like this, it will also hinder your psychic abilities, making you feel too lethargic or low in energy to practice with your gift effectively.

Take care of your aura as you would take care of your physical self. Treat your aura's blockages as you would treat an illness or a broken bone.

How to See Auras

Seeing energy is a much more developed and refined sense. Many have caught a glimpse of it at some point, only to dismiss it as their mind playing tricks on them. They may have seen light, color, or a fuzzy field around a person's outline.

When you first begin to practice seeing auras, it usually begins by seeing what looks like mist and waves. Honing in on colors and other details will take a lot of time and practice for most. Those with a natural proclivity most likely developed their skill in previous incarnations.

There are probably more individuals that can see auras than we realize. People often keep such details about themselves secret, in the fear that they will be labeled as "weird" or "unstable", and will be rejected or judged by their peers. Nonetheless, those who have this ability sometimes put it to good use.

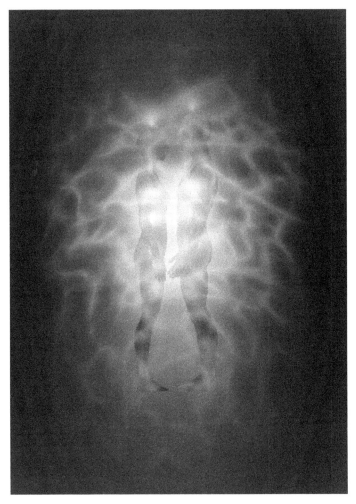

To practice seeing auras, there are certain techniques that can train the eyes to register subtle information.

One such technique involves using the peripheral vision:

- Go into a room with a plant and dim the lights. Ideally the plant will be against a solid, light, neutral wall.

- Look at the plant with your peripheral vision instead of viewing it directly. With repeated practice, a misty outline will appear around the plant.

- After this, you can move onto animals and humans.

Chapter 6 Gain Enlightenment with Spiritual Transcendence Using Meditation

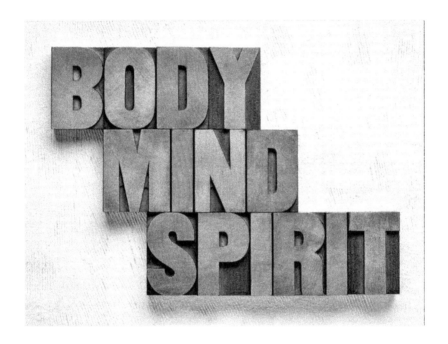

The word Kundalini translates from Sanskrit as "coiled up." This word describes the concept that energy is coiled up at the base of the spine of every person living on earth. It is often depicted as a snake or serpent who lies within the pelvic bowl. As this energy is awakened, the serpent power rises up through the body and all the chakras until it reaches the crown of the head. This coil of energy or snake is the Life-Force, the prana, the divine power that

62

when awakened will lead to an unraveling process, allowing consciousness to shift and become elevated into pure, divine, creation–energy consciousness.

Kundalini yoga is the body practice associated with this energy. The practice of which, along with other meditations, energy, work, and lifestyle choices help the practitioner come into alignment with this divine energy. There are several different yoga practices, each with its own philosophy, mantra and spiritual expression, or goal.

Kundalini Awakening can be very intense and the experience of ascension is different for everyone. It can turn your whole world and life upside-down. You may change your whole lifestyle, or fearlessly start your dream job; you may move to another country to practice your new wholeness and enlightenment in a like-minded community, and you may become a benefactor or a volunteer. Sometimes it can be scary and unpredictable to begin such a journey. It's easy to keep things the way they are, but if you know that you have the power within you to awaken your divine energy, your higher consciousness, and ultimately the source of your primal spark, the energy of creation, why wouldn't you?

There are so many significant benefits to taking this path of transformation for your mind, body, and spirit. Below are some of the advantages of an awakened existence through the process of Kundalini Awakening.

Mind

Overall enhancement of memory and cognitive ability; clear thinking.

Ability to face the uncontrollable and unpredictable ups and downs of life with more peace and tranquility.

Greater mental focus and self-control.

Enhanced senses and perceptions.

Reduction in feelings of anger, shame, guilt, depression, and anxiety.

Self-love and compassion and empathy for others.

Increased or awakened psychic capabilities.

Body
More balanced and healthy function of various body systems including digestion, lymphatic flow, and cardiovascular health.

Stronger and more balanced immune system.

Elimination of bad habits such as smoking, excessive alcohol or drug use, and overeating.

Overall improvement in physical strength.

Increase in energy and vitality.

Can possibly eradicate ongoing or chronic health issues such as irritable bowel syndrome, kidney stones, edema, and skin discoloration due to poor circulation.

Better sleep.

Spirit
Increase in a spiritual connection with self, others, and the Universe.

Higher vibrational frequency in your body's energy to magnetically attract things, situations, and people to you with your thoughts.

Heightened awareness of the flows of energy in all life and matter.

Balanced chakras and inner energies that lead to an overall feeling of alignment and transcendence.

Awakened inner-eye or third eye to promote connection to the divine, experience visions, astral travel, and latent psychic abilities.

Spiritual radiance, bliss, peace, healing, and calm.

These are several of the benefits and of course, there are more. Kundalini awakening is such a gift to the soul, to the individual consciousness and to the realization that we are all connected and have this special opportunity to become more enlightened, evolved, healed, and in tune to our greatest gift of Divine consciousness. The benefits of transformation, enlightenment, and transcendence far outweigh costs. And what is the cost, you may ask. The cost, dear reader, is that you commit yourself to an amazing journey of self-discovery, a path of inner enrichment and an embodiment of feeling one with the Universe.

On achieving enlightenment

Anyone who walks a spiritual path would wonder about achieving enlightenment. In the Christian tradition, this is referred to as heaven. In Buddhism, it is known as Nirvana.

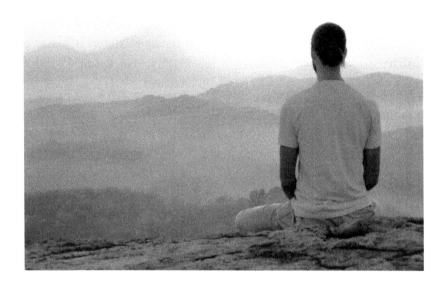

Many other traditions have given it many names, but they all refer to the same thing. You are probably familiar with stories of Buddhists who seek enlightenment. Take, for example, how Siddhartha Gautama Buddha was enlightened while meditating under a tree. There are many other stories of how certain people reached the state of Nirvana or enlightenment.You have to understand that there is no single path towards enlightenment. Hence, you cannot say that you need to be a Buddhist or a Hindu to be enlightened. True enlightenment is open for all, even to a person who has no religion. Unfortunately, it is also true that only a few reach this state of enlightenment. However, do not be discouraged.

As the saying goes, it is not reaching the top of the mountain that matters, the true journey lies in the path itself. But, of course, it would still be a big bonus to be enlightened in this lifetime.

So, is it important to be enlightened? This would depend on your personal belief and preferences. For example, in Buddhism, enlightenment is the way to escape from samsara or the endless cycle of birth and rebirth.

In Christianity, you can be thrown to eternal damnation (hell) for eternity. In other traditions, it is believed that the goal of every human being is to achieve enlightenment. However, there are also people who have realized and accepted that they will not achieve enlightenment in this lifetime. Instead, they explore other venues like engaging in psychic powers, so that they can focus on attaining enlightenment in their next life. Hence, with respect to this matter, you should think about it and make your own reflections. It is only you who can answer it. Do you consider attaining enlightenment important in the current life that you have?

People have many different views about this. For some, enlightenment is the main goal on their spiritual journey. Others do not think enlightenment is important. Many believe that they will not even reach enlightenment in their lifetime.

This is not saying they don't need to do good things. You can be good without ever achieving enlightenment. When Buddha achieved enlightenment, he was a very good person before that happened. He was a very spiritual person. Once he achieved enlightenment, his life got more meaningful and richer. It all depends on you as to whether or not enlightenment is important.

Chapter 7 How to move a manipulate energy

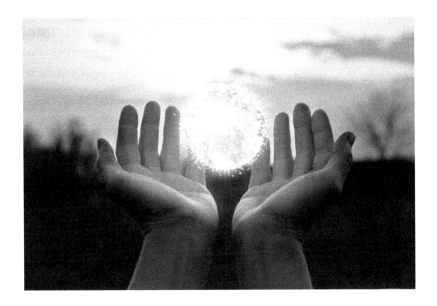

E nergy is an animated and palpable life force-one that all of us can understand in the context of our daily life. We usually attribute our low energy days to either bad food, lack of sleep or even the weather. However, the more significant issue is more complicated than it seems. Our energetic systems might be impacted by emotional, physical and even cognitive blocks that we have picked up from far back into our childhood and which we do not even realize.

Energy & Consciousness

The word is often manipulated into defining it in scientific or even in mystical terms and in the process of wanting to define it, we take out the value or deeper understanding of energy.

All every one of us understands about energy is to stay quiet and rest in ourselves and feel our surroundings. For instance, when we feel present, our energy is rooted, or when we feel repulsion or attraction, we feel energetically charged. When we feel like laughing or crying, we feel energy leaving us. Certain situations and yes, people can deplete our energy or even places. On the flip side, we also cling on to people, situations, and places that fuel our source of energy especially when we feel we are not enough.

Energy can neither be created nor destroyed, but it can be altered. We can speed up or slow down energy, and it can exist in closed systems where this energy can help, or it can even exist in an open system where the energy flows. The energy that is uncontained can cause a fragmented or frenetic system. Likewise, the energy that has depleted can also cause a system to collapse.

Energy, despite its power, is a neutral force. It is basically a consciousness that directs its movement. If we see energy like we see consciousness, then we become more direct with our energy moving towards connection and creation as well as evolution. The less conscious you are, the more energy separates from us.

Blocked Energy

Our mind is open and flexible, and our breath is rhythmic and deep and makes us feel spacious in our body. When we are in our Kundalini flow, we enable ourselves to get into a healthy balance that is between contraction and expansion as well as activation and receptivity.

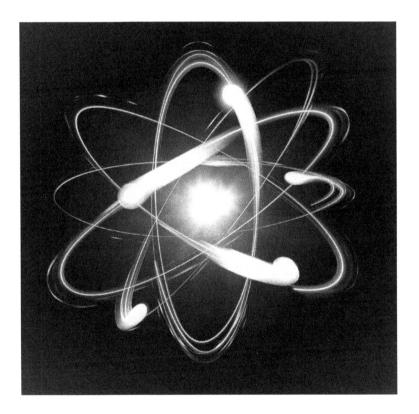

We allow our reasoning, emotions and will to work in partnership with each other and in the process, we create faith in ourselves and often times find ourselves undefended-this is called energy integrity. Energy integrity is usually short-lived, and many people will often describe this energy as stagnant or blocked or even stuck. This is a very narrow-minded thinking all because their breathing, and even their posture is not corrected.

Sensing Energy

Of all things you can first try to do, sensing energy is difficult to accomplish straight away. This is not very common. However, there are techniques that you can do to sense and manipulate energy:

1) Like everything else, close your eyes and start by visualizing your body with all its veins
2) Visualize the veins you see but instead of picturing it red with blood, picture it carrying energy and this can be in any color you relate to. See the energy circling through your body touching each and every nerve.
3) Next, try sensing the vibrations that come while this energy circulates throughout.
4) Focus on a specific body part, such as the arms and tell the energy in your body to course specifically to that area. If you feel or notice any tingling sensation, it is probably successful energy manipulation. Try again on your other arm and then move on to your legs.
5) Once you are done moving the energy around your body, allow the energy to flow back naturally again throughout your body.

Do not be disappointed if you did not get any feeling the first time or even a few times after that. Energy manipulation is not easy, so it takes practice, patience and time.

Programming

The main component of energy manipulation is programming. There are plenty of ways to program, and for different people, different programs work better for them. Programming and energy manipulation work in tandem with each other.

Energy Manipulation and Chakras

Chakras may or may not be useful or even necessary in energy manipulation however the logic here is that energy passes through chakras to it is always important to check your chakra balance and make sure they are not clogged. Energy manipulation may not be successful if you have blocked chakras.

Absorbing Energy

There are plenty of ways to absorb energy. It could be from other people, it can also be from within us. We can also absorb chakras from situations, places, and experiences.

If you want to absorb energy, here is what you can do:

1) Pick a target from which you want to absorb your energy from. It is good to take energy from an inanimate object such as a tree or a flower. This source of energy must not affect the energy that you are receiving from.
2) Concentrate on said object and then try to establish a link between yourself and the object. You can make this a little easier by visualizing a wire connecting you and this object together.
3) Visualize the energy that is flowing from the object towards you. Take only what you need and not anymore.

If you are planning on taking energy from a person, you must always ask for their permission first before attempting to take it. Not asking for permission might result in negative consequences as the energy was obtained unknowingly or without consent, which is why it is encouraged to take energy from inanimate objects.

You can also absorb energy from the situation around you. This is called ambient energy and to retrieve this you simply visualize a link to the energy from where you are standing or sitting in the environment.

Releasing energy is often done only when you feel like you have taken too much of it. All you need to do is do the reverse of the steps described above.

Chapter 8 Chakra Healing

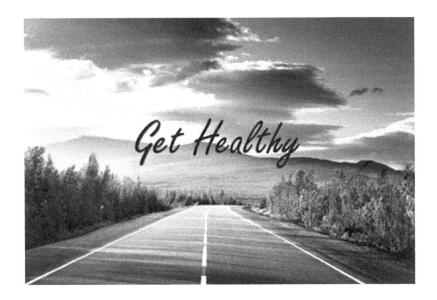

Since you need a healthy chakra system in order to awaken your Kundalini, it is important that you know how to heal them. All of your chakras have a close connection to your physical body. Healthy chakras keep your physical body healthy. One of the easiest ways to keep your chakras healthy is to make sure that you keep your body healthy and fit. This is why regular exercise is important. Exercising is one of the most natural ways to cleanse your chakras.

You do not have to go crazy with your workouts either. Something as simple as walking or jogging is perfect. The most important thing is that you love yourself and your body and shake off all of your negative energy.

Eating healthy is another important part of keeping your chakras healthy. Make sure you consume plenty of vegetables and reduce the number of processed foods you eat. There are some people who say you should avoid dairy and meat products as well. You do not have to be vegan, but try to choose greens and healthy foods as much as possible. If you are not already a healthy eater, you can become healthier by gradually adding in healthier foods and slowly eliminating unhealthy foods.

Making positive lifestyle changes are also important. If you are a smoker, you should stop. You do not have to go cold turkey, just slowly reduce the number of cigarettes you smoke each day until you reach zero. Also, if you are a heavy drinker, try to reduce the number of alcoholic beverages you consume. The more physically healthy your body is, the more energized and cleansed your chakra system will become.

The truth of the matter is that it is hard to be healthy, especially when you are used to following so many unhealthy habits. It does not have to be this way forever. Be happy that you have experienced these habits and learn from them. Start to make small changes and think about doing things that are good for your body. There are some traditions that impose strict rules on their followers. Some go so far as to eliminate all animal products and alcohol from the diet in order to awaken their Kundalini.

The great thing is unless you do follow a tradition that imposes these, all you need to do is follow a healthier lifestyle. It is also important to act in a positive manner. This can be tough when you first start making these changes, but soon they will become second nature. Eventually, you will become lost in how amazing you feel with your new healthy habits.

So, how do you heal chakras easily and naturally? Remember that the chakras are connected to your physical body. By maintaining a healthy body, you also get to empower the chakras. Therefore, to keep your chakras healthy, you should keep your body healthy. The problem comes when you consider how to maintain a healthy physical body. Many people say that you should eat chicken and poultry products to gain protein and other "healthy" nutrients. However, as far as spirituality is concerned, especially if you want to awaken your Kundalini, it is advised that you stay away from eating meat and poultry products. Instead, you should observe a vegan or vegetarian diet. It is also worth noting that there are studies that have proven that eating meat can cause lots of diseases, including diabetes and cancer, among others. If you find it hard to stay away from meat and poultry, then at least try to minimize your consumption of the said products.

Doing regular exercise is also encouraged. In fact, exercising is one of the body's natural ways to remove negative energies from your system. You do not need to engage in a heavy workout. A light workout like walking or jogging would be enough. Simply put, everything that is good for the physical body is also good for your chakras. Indeed, this is another reason for you to be healthy.

Heal your chakras through meditation

The best way to work on your chakras is through meditation. Of course, this does not mean that adopting a healthy lifestyle is no longer important. Remember that when you treat or heal something, you also need to look into the main cause or source of the problem. Hence, if you know that it is your lifestyle that is continuously bringing you unhealthy and dirty energies, then you need to make some adjustments.

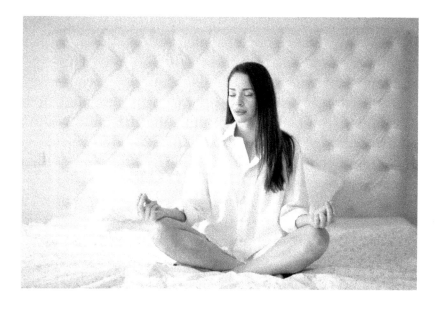

It is true that all meditation practices help to develop the chakras. In fact, even the simple breathing meditation that we have discussed also helps with cleansing your chakras of negative energies. However, there are certain meditations that work directly to achieve a specific objective. As you go through this book, you will learn different meditation that techniques that not only enhance your overall system and chakras but also specialize in certain parts of your spiritual or energy body. For now, here is an excellent meditation that can help you cleanse and heal your chakras:

Assume a meditative position and relax. Visualize a powerful ray of light descending from heaven and moving down into your crown chakra, charging it with immense power. See and feel your crown chakra being cleansed and recharged. Do not stop until you see and feel that your crown chakra is fully cleansed and is radiating with powerful light. Now, send this divine energy down to the Ajna or third eye chakra. Allow the powerful ray of divine light to cleanse and charge your Ajna chakra.

Once you are satisfied, send the energy to the next chakra, which is the throat chakra. Allow this divine energy to cleanse and supercharge your throat chakra. Next, let the ray of light descend down to your heart chakra. See and feel as your heart chakra shines brilliantly, free from all dirt and negativity. Now, allow the ray for light to descend down to your solar plexus chakra. Allow the light to cleanse and charge this chakra. Send the light further down to your sacral chakra, and feel how the light empowers this chakra. Finally, send the divine light down to your root chakra. Feel yourself being more stable and grounded. Allow this ray of light to fully cleansed and charge your root chakra.

Once you have charged and cleansed all your chakras, see and feel all the seven main chakras radiating powerfully and full of brilliance. Visualize the divine ray of light slowly fade away. Say a short prayer and thank God or the universe for cleansing and healing you. Enjoy this moment of divine bliss and peace.

When you are ready to return to ordinary consciousness, gently move your fingers and toes, and slowly open your eyes.

The meditation technique above is one of the best ways to empower and heal the chakras through meditation. You are free to make adjustments or modifications if you want.

The important thing is to charge and purify your chakras. The said ray of light can be visualized in any way you want. You can see it having the same color as the chakra being cleansed and charged, but you can also just use white light to make the visualization simpler. After all, the color white is the color of Akasha. As such, it possesses all the colors.

Chapter 9 Secret meditation techniques with awakening kundalini

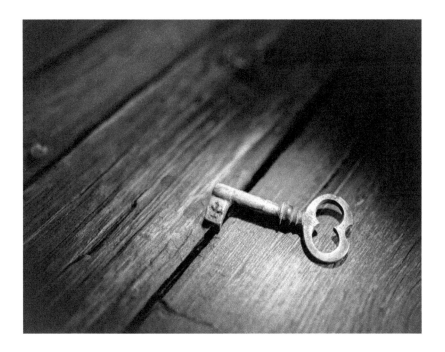

Mantra Meditation

Mantra meditation is probably one of the oldest and commonly used meditation techniques in the world. What is a mantra? A mantra is a sound, word, or syllable that functions as your point of focus in meditation. A good example of a mantra is the mantra OM.

The mantra OM has been used by spiritual masters and meditators around the world for centuries. It is said to be the first sound in the universe. Indeed, it has a rich history. It is also the mantra that is commonly used by Buddhists and Hindus.

The purpose of the mantra is to help still the mind. If you allow the untrained mind to be as it is, then you will be bombarded with so many thoughts that it would be hard for you to meditate. When you use a mantra, you limit your mind to a single thought (the mantra).

Think of your mantra as the vehicle that you use in a spiritual pilgrimage. By focusing on and becoming one with your mantra, you will be taken to a deeper state of consciousness. The whole meditation practice itself is the journey, and your mantra is the vehicle.

For this meditation, let us use the mantra OM. It is important to note that when you say the mantra OM, you should give it a resonating sound. You can find many videos on YouTube on how to do this. This is the correct way to recite a mantra, as it could help you reach a higher state of consciousness. Let us now proceed to the meditation proper:

Assume a meditative position. Relax. Gently start to recite your mantra aloud. For this meditation, we will be using the mantra OM. The mantra OM is the first sound ever made in the universe, and many spiritual gurus have made use of this mantra. By using the same mantra, you also get to connect yourself to these spiritual gurus and masters. Place all your focus on the mantra OM, and pay no attention to any other thought or any emotions that may arise during this meditation. Be one with the mantra OM. Nothing in this universe exists but the mantra OM. Continue to recite the mantra. Relax and let go.

When you are ready to return to your physical body, simply bring your attention back to your physical body, gently move your fingers and toes, and open your eyes with a smile.

You can, of course, do this meditation technique for a longer period, but doing it for only five minutes will also be fine. Remember that when thoughts arise in the mind (monkey mind), you should simply ignore them. Do not use a year kind of force.

Affirmation meditation

These days, many people talk about the use of affirmations. For example, when you are feeling afraid, you tell yourself, "I am strong and courageous." The secret to using an affirmation effectively is to recite it when you are in a meditative state. This is because the subconscious mind is more susceptible to suggestions when you are doing meditation.

Assume a meditative position and relax. Breathe in gently, and out. Think of a happy memory and absorb the positive energy of that memory. Now, start to recite your affirmation. Your affirmation is your mantra. Be one with it. Do this for as long as you are comfortable or until you have this strong feeling that your desire has completely been communicated to your subconscious. Remember that you are just affirming something, so you do not need to use force. Have faith. Affirm and let go.

It is also suggested that you should avoid using different affirmations. Only use one affirmation at a time. Hence, do not move on to another objective unless the first or previous objective has not yet manifested in the physical realm. Be patient.

Positive energy recharge

Assume a meditative posture and relax. Now, think of a happy event or memory. Re-experience this happy memory in your mind.

If you want, you can also create your own happy event. I want you to fully submerge yourself in this thought and experience it as if it were happening at this very moment. Do you feel the joy and the love in your life?

Now, think about another happy event. Once again, experience this event/memory as much as you can. Use all of our senses. Look around you and pay attention to every person and every being around you. Breathe in the positive energy of this memory.

You can end the exercise here, but you can also move on to another happy memory as many times as you want. Once you are ready to return to your physical body, simply think of your physical body, gently move your fingers, and open your eyes with a smile.

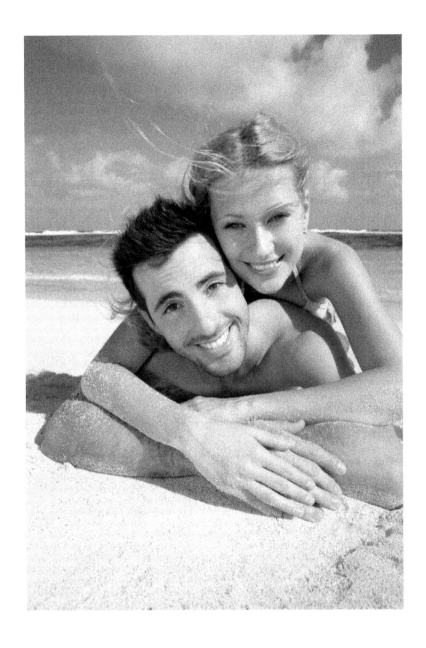

Waterfall cleansing meditation

Assume a meditative posture and relax. Visualize yourself sitting under a waterfall. Feel the cold and clean water as it falls on your body. As you do, see and feel that the water not only cleanses your physical body but also cleanses all the dirt on your aura and your soul.

You are getting cleaner and cleaner every second. See yourself shining in white dazzling brilliance. Continue to cleanse yourself in this way until you are shining brightly and fully cleansed.

Whole body breathing meditation

Assume a meditative position and relax completely. Now, as you breathe in, visualize that it is your whole body that breathes in prana. See and feel the vital energy entering through every pore of your body. You are to visualize yourself as a sponge that hungrily sucks in prana all around you. You can visualize the prana in any way you want. For starters, you can imagine the universal energy as white light. Breathe in this powerful universal energy through the whole body and charge yourself with it. Continue to do this until you are fully charged with energy.

There is also what is known as the cleansing breath. It is simply the opposite wherein you breathe out negative energies. If you want, you can combine this with whole body breathing. Breathe in positive energy and then breathe out all negative energies from your system. It is usually advised to limit it to 7 cycles. You can then increase the number of cycles as you get used to it. One cycle is composed of one inhalation followed by an exhalation.

Cold water cleanse

Place a glass of cold water in front of you. Now, think about all the things that bother you and give you stress. Whisper or shout them at the cold water. Pass the negativity to the water. Since cold water has a strong magnetizing element, it will receive whatever you send it. Be emotional if you want, the important thing is to let all the negativity out and be passed to the water.

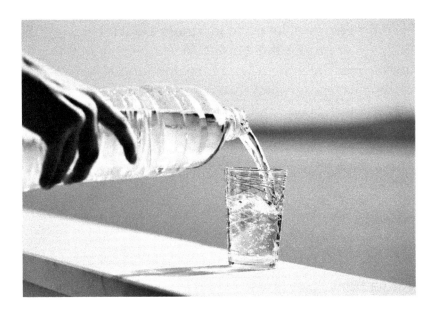

When you are done, you will be feeling much better, as if you have removed a bad load – which you actually did. Now, throw away the water. It should be noted that you should never drink the water that has absorbed your negative energies. Just throw it away or have it go down the drain. It is also not advised to drink using the cup that you used for this exercise, as it has become a home for negativity. However, should you need to use it; you can easily cleanse the cup by washing it with saltwater as you visualize the negative energies being washed away completely.

Blessing meditation

Assume a meditative position and relax. Raise your hands slightly in a blessing position with your palms facing outwards. Visualize the person whom you want to bless standing in front of you. Now, imagine a white or golden light coming from above and entering the top of your head. This is the energy of love and kindness. Let it fill your whole being. Now, project this energy to the person standing in front of you. Bless them with love and kindness. See them receive this energy and becoming happier and happier every second. If you want, you can visualize another person and repeat the process. You can do this as many times as you want.

Although you can use your personal energy, doing so can drain you in the end, so it is good to draw energy from the universe.

Healing light

Assume a meditative position. Now, visualize a white ray of light from the heaven, and send it to the ailing body part. This ray of light is pure healing energy of the universe. It heals anything and everything that it touches. Allow the energy to accumulate in your chosen area. Feel its power. Continue to charge the said part with the pure energy of healing.

You can also fill your whole body with healing energy. It is important that you believe in the power of what you are doing. Firmly believe that that the ray of light and heal anything. Energy healing like Reiki and Pranic Healing are just one of the schools of healing that make use of prana for healing. Indeed, prana can heal all forms of diseases, but you need to practice your skills for you to be good at it.

Healing is one of the most important applications of prana and psychic abilities. Unfortunately, only a few are truly able to do it properly. If you practice enough, then you can be an effective healer.

Whole body healing

Assume a meditative position and relax. See and feel yourself sitting on the shore. Watch as the waves come and go. The sea before you is full of healing energy. Now, stand up and walk slowly towards the water. Allow the waves stop touch your feet. Do you feel the healing power of water? Continue to step towards the sea and allow the water level to go up your knees, see and feel the healing energy of water enter your feet and your knees, charging you with powerful healing energy. Now, step further into the water and let it wet your body to the waist level. Feel the healing energy of water penetrate your body from the waist down. Again, step forward and let the water bathe you completely up to your neck. Feel the cold water and its powerful healing energy bathing you. Spend more time in this position. You are about to soak your whole body; when you do, you will be filled with the pure healing energy of water. Now, take another step forward. Your whole body is now submerged in water. Since you are in the astral plane, you would not have any problem with breathing. Continue to move forward and go deeper and deeper into the sea.

You are filled with nothing but healing energy. Feel all the negativity in your system being cleansed and washed away. You are pure and clean. You can stay in this state for as long as you want.

When you are ready to end the meditation, simply take a step back until you reach the shore. Watch the healing waves as they come and go, and thank the water spirits. Think of your physical body and desire yourself to go back to your physical body. Gently move your fingers and toes, and open your eyes with a smile.

The element of water is associated with healing. Allowing this element to fill your body is an effective way to cleanse your system and heal diseases. Of course, this technique has to be practiced for you to be good at it. You must have the firm determination and certainty that the water is a strong healing agent and that it actually heals you when you fill yourself with this element in your meditation.

Take note that these meditation sessions can take longer than 30 minutes. When meditating, time is of learning importance. The important thing is the quality of your meditation. After all, remember that the more that you go deeper into a trance state, the more that time will not exist. It is also worth noting that the key to mastery of meditation is to do it repeatedly and regularly. Do not be discouraged even if you feel nothing the first time you try to meditate. It only means that you need to practice it more. If you persist in these practices, rest assured that you would soon reap the wonderful benefits of meditation.

Chapter 10 How to mastery Kundalini

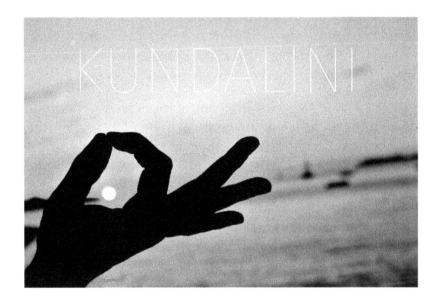

Now that you understand that your Kundalini is a reservoir of spiritual energy and that it gives you aliveness, purpose and passion, let's look at how you can begin to awaken this energy. Kundalini is probably the most sensual energy you could ever imagine.

Once you go through a Kundalini awakening you feel as if you have been healed. You will have the feeling of being able to change anything and everything that is in your life. You will have access to an unlimited well of energy, knowledge and the sensation that your soul will not die.

As soon as you have awakened your Kundalini, you will begin to see the spiritual truth behind all things. You will start to see everything, yourself, people you meet and the world, as part of the greater Divine. You are able to realize God is in everything; you communicate with all and understand it to be an intelligent Conscious Energy that helps to support you in everything that you want to do in the world. The things that you communicate with also contain this enlightened consciousness.

Probably one of the most interesting aspects of a Kundalini awakening is what will happen when it works into relationships you have with other people. You will be able to connect, love and trust them purely because the higher intelligence is found everywhere. You will be able to let go of judgments, get rid of any existing blocks, drop any resistance to love and fear of intimacy. Once your mind is consumed with the Kundalini energy, you will feel amazing and powerful because it clears away everything that is blocking you from being your true self with others.

With the awakening you will drop that veil that prevents you from seeing the truth of the world. You will enter a world to your spiritual self, true love, abundance and become one with the Divine that is in everything around you. As the Kundalini awakens, it will move up your spine. It can feel warm or tingling. These sensations are the energy purifying you and will bring you to the highest conscious state.

You will receive an expanded energy state, blissful love and cosmic thinking. You will be able to comprehend reality and you will know what complete freedom from suffering is like and the possibility for enlightenment. You will constantly feel happy and everything you do, the choices you make, will always be the best.

One of the best aspects of awakening your Kundalini is the healing energy that you will receive. You will soon be able to heal yourself and others that are willing and open. Kundalini power is fierce and it has no limitations. The energy that you will have coursing through you will be contagious to everybody that comes in contact with you. People around you will leave feeling more free, happier and higher. By being yourself, you will naturally enlighten the world around you. This is something that you can really get thrilled about.

An essential part of being able to experience a full awakening is how committed you are to your spiritual path. How devoted are you to seeing and feeling the divine that lives in everything and everyone? How much do you want to let in trust and get rid of doubt? A good way of figuring out how devoted you .are is to see how you feel around people that typically make you suffer. If you are devoted to something, you will practice compassion towards everybody, even the ones that cause you pain. You are able to relax your body which is what Kundalini needs to be able to move. When you are totally devoted to being able to relax in this connection, you will naturally be able to connect with the universe and awaken your Kundalini.

It is a good thing to know that Kundalini lives within you; all you have to do is wake it up. If you were to wake her up without knowing the proper way to do so, you may end up disrupting your typical reality. This can end up being negative or positive; it all depends on how you perceive it. If you have the correct foundation you will have a rather enjoyable experience.

To start your awakening journey, begin by practicing a special Kundalini meditation every day. There are several ways to awaken your Kundalini, but the most popular is to breathe in a golden light all the way up and down your spine as much as you are able to all day. This can be done when you are watching TV, resting, eating, cooking, standing in line, driving, you can do it anytime because you are constantly breathing.

The next step is to accept any issues, energy, people, or thoughts that you are trying to stay away from. These things are there to teach you and a person who has been through an awakening will run to these types of things to explore their meaning and find a deeper compassion that is hiding within. Kundalini will give you limitless amounts of happiness.

The next thing would be to ask yourself what you think is necessary to achieve the emotion or feeling that you most desire to have. What is out there that can help you feel at peace? I would suggest stop running and turn your focus to the connection you have with the divine that already lives inside you. This is living at the base of your spine.

It is important to know that this awakening can be the best thing that has ever happened to you if you are fully devoted, or it can be the worst that that has ever happened because you aren't fully devoted. It depends on how you look at it; is it "for you" or "to you". This type of a paradigm shift will depend on your attachment to your ego.

When you are able to take that step past your ego is the biggest part of opening all the doors in you for Kundalini to flow. To be able to get rid of your ego you have to honor this: you are an infinite soul that can never die. You have to truly believe that you are not just a physical body, instead you have a spiritual immortal. Perspective is an important part of being able to handle Kundalini rushing through you. The more inclusive you are on your perspective of your spiritual being, the easier it will become for you to accept the energy of Kundalini.

There are two more factors that play into being able to awaken your Kundalini. First, how sensually and sexually open you are. Second, how open you are to a spiritual transformation. If you have an open sensual and sexual energy flow with the source, then the pathway is already paved to receive the energy from Kundalini. This does not just mean your sex center, but every center that lives up your spine. The bottom three, solar plexus down, is the foundation you need to build. It needs to be relaxed and solid for your Kundalini to rise up through.

When you awaken you Kundalini it can feel like you have tapped into a million watts while your body can only hold 100 watts. This is way you need to prepare yourself to be able to easily accept the million watts with ease. Daily meditation can help you to receive all of this energy. Your body will become opened enough to be able to receive this healing energy from the universe.

This is a lifelong commitment, so start today. Begin by loving how your life is at this moment and start being aware, awake and living in the moment. Treat your body gently and love it as it is. Listen to yourself and give it what it needs. This includes have a good diet, bathing, exercising and treating it like it's sacred. There are likely several mental and emotional blocks within your body that is attached to your ego that causes some limited beliefs. These blocks will interfere with your awakening.

Definitely do not try to force your awakening. If you try to push it through any sexual blocks, you will likely experience pain. This is telling you to stop and work on emotion healing. Pain is the body's way of telling you to slow down, listen, be silent, heal and relax. Be gentle on yourself and continue to do your daily practices. You will end up having better health, energy and sex.

When you open your Kundalini you will find creative energy and you will want to become more conscious, alive and healed. This will make your life full of more joy, love and gratitude than you have ever felt before.

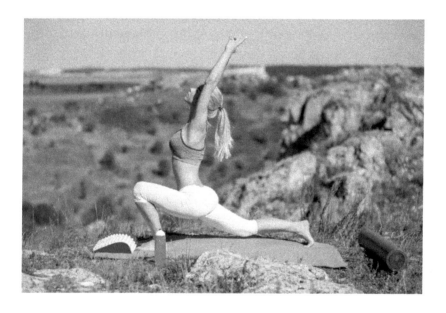

It is important to know that the universe will never give you anything that you are not able to handle, or that you need, on some level. If you have a severely blocked Kundalini and you find that sex is painful, this pain means that you have trauma that is locked within the cells and wounds that are trying to be fixed. BE GENTLE! The golden rule of Kundalini awakening is, be gentle and heal your wounds.

You will find a lot of people say that awakening makes you go crazy, or that there is a ton of energy and that you feel out of control, this is just your ego falling away. Kundalini is a fire that will burn away your ego and you will become liberated to follow your spiritual path. This is how you become purified from suffering in the past, present and future. That is what makes Kundalini so amazing.

Opening your heart to love is a secret to experiencing a blissful awakening. When you have love, everything you experience is amazing. Ease yourself into meditation and allow love to guide you.

Your ego is what makes you want instant gratification and results. That is why it's hard to stick with a weight loss regimen because you want it to work overnight. If you allow your ego to rule your awakening, you will only cause a delay in your awakening.

If you are completely and truly devoted to your spiritual focus, then you will have a connection to love and then all you have to do is surrender to it.

Your Kundalini energy wants to be able to travel up your spine and through your head to give you a direct connection to the divine. It's designed this way so you can carve you own spiritual path so you can see where you need to travel. By performing a simple Kundalini meditation, you will automatically feel an energy expansion and will cause tingling sensations in your spine that will give you enjoyable energy waves.

By making the choice to go through an awakening is one of the best gifts that you can give yourself. You will love other people, and you will be able to enjoy life a lot more.

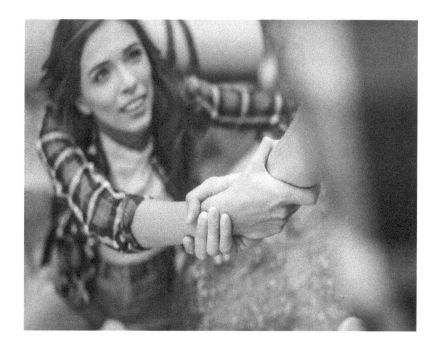

Each sight, touch, smell and taste will have a deeper connection than ever before. It is definitely a higher level of living.

Tips for Your Awakening Process

The awakening process, whether performed through spiritual discipline, or by accident, can cause challenges for you. It's like your body has been amped to 110-220 wiring and as the appliance, you haven't learned how to adapt your body to it. It is very rare for you to go through an awakening before you have completed months and possibly years, of clearing.

This energy's goal is to bring you together with your universal self, non-self, or with the peace that is passed through understanding.

Some scripture refers to Kundalini as a goddess, they called her Shakti, which can awaken and runs through the body all the way through the top of the head to connect with the God Shiva, her lover. This represents universal consciousness.

During this journey your self-identification, illusions and beliefs that relate to your current personality are dissolved away. You may end up feeling like you don't belong in this world. You are instead moving towards a vastness of the entire world.

The clearing is said to be a purification process, or, according to the Hindu, you will release your samskaras and vrittis.

Samskaras refers to the need to work out problems for past lives, or the consequences of things that have happened in your present life. Vrittis refers to the movement of your thoughts and mind. There are several practices that work to overcome and calm the vrittis activity.

You are a spirit that lives in a physical body. The cells of your body are similar to a hologram and they contain memories from everything that has ever happened to you.

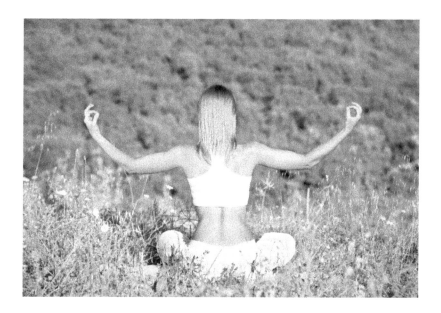

When the energy moves through and transforms the body, the areas with contractions, memory, pain, or energy will react to the change. This is when you will have feelings of rushes, vibrations, heat, jerking, pain and other such phenomena during an awakening. Sometimes these movements are associated with a chakra as it is opened, which is just another way of saying that as a pain is release, new possibilities will emerge.

Each person deals and carries their pain in several different ways, just like you live your life in a way different than me and so there are several different ways that you can respond to the new energy. If you suffer from physical problems that come from an old injury, you may notice that area to be extra sensitive. If you consume an unhealthy diet, or your lifestyle puts you in a toxic emotional energy, this can cause you to be more susceptible to difficulties. If you have suffered any kind of abuse, or you have a history of drug use or alcoholism, your body may be hard to awaken because it is trying to clear out all of the past memories. If you have a tendency to fight against things and you like to have full control, you will find that the process is a lot hard because of your resistance.

You may feel the energy as intense and coarse, but it's very rarely painful. Typically fear and trying to stop it, will be the cause of the pain. If you experience a lot of bodily movement, lay down a couple of times during the day and allow the energy to spread throughout you and allow it to remove the blockages that don't belong to you and what needs to be released at that moment in time. This typically takes about 20 minutes and then you will be able to relax. This needs to be done if you work where you are more exposed to negative energy or pain from others like therapeutic or healing work, or if you work where there is a lot of alcohol consumed, or in hospitals. If you continue to have constant physical pain, it may be in your best interest to be medically evaluated.

Find out what it is your body actually wants to eat. A lot of the time you will find that you are in need of a major dietary shift like eating smaller meals, avoid red meat, going on a plant based diet and give up alcohol and drugs. If you struggle with a persistent problem with your energy, start doing detective work to figure out what it is that can be causing your problem.

Pay attention to your belly and heart and not so much in your head. Use practices that help to center you into the present. The best options are devotional practices like heart centered meditation or chanting. These help to open you to experience your deeper self, the eternal self. Start creating more connections with other people. It is also a good idea to start volunteering either for nature or animal organizations; this can help your awakening to be more balanced. You may even find it comforting to call upon an image of an ally like a symbol, saint, teacher, goddess, or god. You can also imagine a golden light surrounding you. There are some that have found success in talking to Kundalini as a Goddess. These are different types of archetypal energies that can help your psyche as it travels through several challenges during your change.

Practice things that help you to be more open. Things like long walks, movement processes, acupressure, dance, Tai Chi, yoga, or anything else that you find yourself drawn to. If you are not sure of what fits you best, start experimenting and find what feels best to you. Your body is what carries you and grounds your spirit. No matter how realized you are, you will be living in your body for many years to come. The more you take care of it, the better options you will have to express your realizations. Somebody who is sick or dying can be a complete and beautiful expression of the divine as much as a healthy person. Poor health does not keep you from being able to be enlightened. People that have sat with the dying have said that as earthy attachments let go, more light will shine through. You should not see this as advocacy for asceticism. While you are alive, having a body that is flexible and open can accomplish the exact same thing and without all the distraction and pain. It is also useless to discipline your body by over doing physical activity. You have to find that mid line that brings together the body and the spirit.

Know when you wake up that you do not know what is going to happen and be excited to find out things as they happen. Instead of constantly being in control and worrying about things, just be present in the moment and be ready for whatever may come up with the intention of handling it the best you can. The things that happen during an awakening will be completely unpredictable and will pass, as long as you simply notice them and you do not try to control it or fight it.

You will sometimes experience psychic openings, energetic swings, emotional swings and several other shifts that will be unfamiliar to you. Just observe what happens. Do not think you have to fix these changes. This will eventually pass.

If you ever experienced any serious trauma in your past and you did not go through therapy, it would be extremely useful to release any pain you have associated with these memories that may come up. People that successfully went through good therapy before they started their awakenings did not have as many difficulties. Therapy gives you the skills to express witness and release so that you can move past the problem. The therapist does not have to understand what Kundalini is, as long as they accept that it is part of the process you are going through. What you are more interested in then is to learn how to release emotions related to your past. Make sure that you find a therapist that is compassionate and experienced and views your spirituality as support and motivation to work through your healing.

The process of awakening is your chance to awaken you true nature. Some may be able to wake first and then go through their Kundalini awakening; others have to go through the Kundalini awakening first. This arising happens to help clear things out. The waking up process helps you to realize that the person is looking out of your eyes, living with your senses, hearing what you think and being present in everything, bad or good, is seen and remembered.

Stop being around people and places that create pain in your life. You will probably become more sensitive when you awaken your Kundalini. You will find it harder to handle the energy in large discount stores, nightclubs, or at competitive and tense family gatherings.

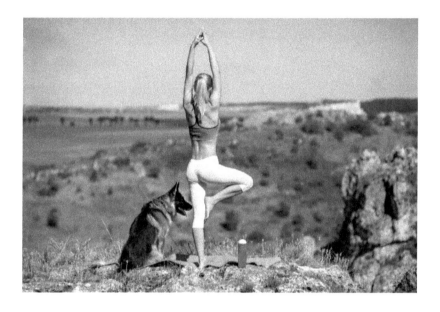

It is perfectly okay to put yourself first and create extra quiet time, more close friendships and possibly a new job, if you find the old one becoming more stressful. You do not ever have to prove anything by making yourself do things you do not want to do. You have to rediscover who you are and what makes you comfortable and what feels natural. Live authentically.

You may realize you have new creative needs, which gives you a wonderful chance to express yourself. Garden, paint, sculpt, dance, write, draw, any of these are perfect ways to nurture yourself and ease your way through the psychic changes. Get yourself an awakened teacher to spend time with. For most, meditation will become a very intrinsic part of your life.

The awakened teacher can help to convey peace to you and allow you to sit in your true nature's silence. Your awakened teacher can have sort of spiritual persuasion or none at all. They do not even have to be interested in Kundalini.

The important thing is that they show compassion and tolerance for everybody that they work with. You will learn the art of being able to sit and be and you will discover the cure for the suffering in your life. With some time you will find the complaints of the body and mental activity will just fall away and you will find a deep understanding to arise. This will give you a sense of invitation, freshness, openness and completion of your greater self's expression. Once you have completed your awakening you will no longer have any doubt that it was the right thing. Where you will go from there, you won't know. You will just surrender to change.

Ways through which awakening or unraveling can help you.

Health benefits – Despite popular perception, awakening Kundalini is not rocket science. It is not child's play either; with practice and effort, awakening your Kundalini is achievable. This energy is known to be powerful when it comes to preventing, treating, and managing several health conditions. Awakened Kundalini energy is known to be effective against indigestion, gastric troubles, and tumors. In some cases, it might also help fight against deadly diseases such as AIDS (in its final stages). This energy may also be utilized against internal ulcers.

Enhanced intuition and psychic abilities—Although Kundalini isn't primarily meant for increasing psychic abilities or intuition, in its awakened form, it blesses the practitioner with enhanced ESP or Extra Sensory Perception, high intuition, and increased psychic powers as wonderful byproducts.

Heightened focus and concentration—From the mental perspective, awakened Kundalini energy can lead to enhanced concentration and focus. The Ajna chakra, which is also referred to as the third eye according to ancient Hindu yogic philosophy, is closely linked with our concentration abilities and focus. When our Kundalini energy awakens, it cleanses, heals, and balances all seven chakras of our body (including the brow or Ajna chakra) to award us with better concentration and focus.

The practitioner becomes a better person—The most significant aspect of awakened Kundalini is that you become more aware, mindful, and conscious. You feel a greater sense of purpose while living. While we may otherwise simply be existing and going about our daily life, awakened Kundalini helps us live (not merely exist) by being more aware of our thoughts, actions, choices, and feelings.

By becoming more present and mindful of people, things, emotions, and situations around us, we invariably become more compassionate human beings. You will learn to perceive things in the right perspective while being able to decipher the truth/facts clearly in all that you experience through your senses. Healed and balanced chakras— Awakened Kundalini has the power to cleanse and balance all seven chakras of the body, which in turn removes psychological and mental blockages, thus making us more compassionate, creative, purposeful, determined, positive, loving, and successful beings.

Signs and Symptoms of Awakened Kundalini Energy?

Beginners often ask how we can determine if our Kundalini energy has truly awakened or not. Here are some experiences and signs that can signify the arising of the Kundalini force. A blissful tingling sensation along our spinal path as the prana (life) force energy manifests its natural chakra healing and balancing act. You will feel a deep sense of balance, peace, healing, and positivity.

Transcendent and inexplicable mystical visions and other profoundly spiritual experiences.

An enlightened and heightened state of consciousness.

Effortless access to one's deep, inner realms of intuition.

Intense mental imagery of deep and profound personal, emotional, and spiritual significance.

An innate feeling of being one with all forms of life.

Inexplicable out-of-body sensations and experiences.

A more purposeful life with a new sense of meaning.

A complete cathartic release of the multilayered psychological baggage of repressed feelings, thoughts, and emotions.

Chapter 11 Improve health, quality of life, and your emotions and enjoy with the benefits

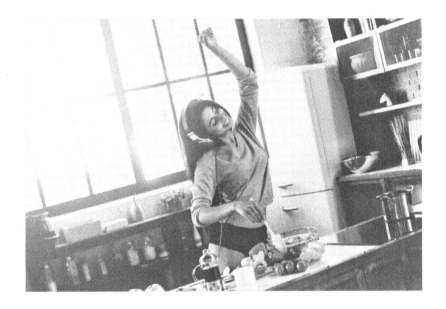

B elieve it or not, your diet has a major impact on Kundalini energy. What you fuel your body with is a form of energy in and of itself. Not only does it provide you with physical energy, but it also works together with your aura and other non-physical energy. It truly does impact you on many different levels. If you want to have a powerful impact on your Kundalini and support it in the best way possible, be sure to pay attention to your diet and what you are eating.

Adjusting Your Diet for Kundalini Awakening

Many people believe that to promote a healthy spiritual flow that you need to be eating a vegetarian or vegan diet. With Kundalini, this is not believed to be necessary. However, it is important that you learn to adjust your diet to suit your body's changing needs. As your spiritual energy changes, your physical body will typically desire to change what it consumes as well. Those who are awakening or who have awakened already tend to avoid eating any foods that introduce unhealthy energies into the body.

Common things that you will likely feel naturally drawn to avoid when you are awakening include things like: alcohol, recreational drugs, red meat, sugar, and excessive chemicals such as the preservatives they put in convenience meals.

You may begin to find yourself wanting or even craving more water, organic whole foods like vegetables and fruits, fish and poultry, or otherwise. Some people may even find themselves naturally being drawn to releasing meats of all varieties and instead pursue a vegetarian or vegan diet. That is perfectly fine, too. The idea here is to listen to your body and what your body wants, as opposed to trying to eat a diet that has been manufactured for you by someone else. Only you know what you need. Following these natural requests from your body will have a major impact on your ability to feel your best and allow your Kundalini energy to flow fluidly.

Listening to Your Body

Your body is already well aware of what it needs to survive and thrive. As you are right now, it is likely that your body has been consuming foods that would keep it comfortable amidst a high-stress lifestyle that may have involved many difficult or painful emotions. This is natural, especially in the Western world where emotional self-care is less popular than in other cultures around the world.

Learning to listen to your body takes some time. Additionally, you may find yourself realizing that as you awaken more, your body needs change.

They may even change beyond diet, encouraging you to exercise differently, use different body care products, or even rest at different times. Being able to really tune into what your body needs is a powerful practice that can truly help you so much in your awakening.

As you grow used to communicating with your body, recognizing what it needs and what it no longer wants becomes significantly easier.

You can begin to intuitively recognize anytime something is causing your body to feel sluggish, slow, or otherwise "off." You can also begin to recognize anytime your body feels empowered, high energy, and positive.

Naturally, you will want to begin practicing more of what makes you feel good and less of what does not. This is how you can intuitively support your body and begin using diet, exercise, and overall physical wellbeing to promote and support your Kundalini awakening and balancing.

Ayurveda Diet and Kundalini
One form of diet that does seem to regularly find itself incorporated in Kundalini awakening and energy is Ayurveda.

Ayurveda is a traditional Hindu system of medicine that uses diet, herbs, and yogic breathing to promote physical, mental, and spiritual wellbeing.

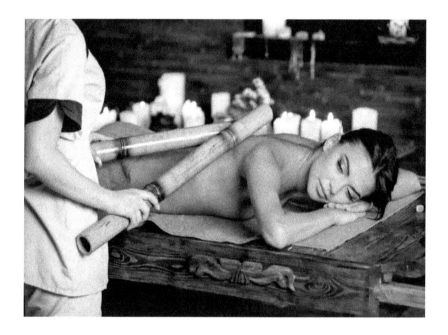

Seeing a professional Ayurvedic practitioner who can assess your unique body type and provide you with advice on how to balance your energies through diet can be powerful. This practice can help you use your diet as a tool to further awaken your energies and thrive, allowing you to feel your best as often as possible. It is a highly recommended tool to use when you are performing your Kundalini awakening, and even when you are balancing your energies.

Health Within Food

It is essential for us to cleanse our human body for our mind and soul to indeed grow and strengthen. We have discussed the dangers of chemicals and other toxins that find their way into our foods through modern processing and food preservation techniques.

Many of our fruits and vegetables are under the influence of harmful pesticides and genetic modification that can and will cause damage to our physical forms. Switching to sources of food that are more reliable will pay off significantly in the end, giving us the right nutrients we need without the harmful side effects of human intervention during the growing process.

Even the meats that we consume daily, if not gathered from high-quality sources, will significantly affect our physical and spiritual lives. The human body is a living thing that requires careful nurturing and guidance for it to thrive and grow to its full potential. Many individuals have resorted to even growing their own vegetable and fruit gardens to guarantee the quality of their food while entirely excluding the use of harmful chemicals.

Many different grocery outlets provide a wide array of organic and healthy foods for us to choose from, allowing us a reprieve from the processed foods that are commonly sold within the larger chains. There are also usually local farmers and stores in smaller towns that offer high-quality organic foods.

Just about all processed foods can have some adverse effect on the human body; this is why the Paleo Diet is commonly used in the practice of Kundalini Awakening. This diet is dedicated to providing humans with foods that they would naturally eat. These foods make it easier for our bodies to process and digest so that we can take more nutrients from our meals and provide our bodies with the proper energy they need. We must keep the mechanics of our body running smoothly if we are to achieve a sense of inner peace and spiritual growth.

Fast food restaurants provide humans with fatty high-processed foods that do nothing but inflict harm upon our pineal gland and our digestive system. While this form of eating can sometimes be convenient, the long-term effects that they have on our physical bodies are entirely negative. Bright candies and drinks are fused with harmful chemicals and dyes that will inflict harm upon our physical form. These colorful dyes infect our brains with dozens of toxins that hinder our capability to grow mentally and spiritually, sometimes even causing horrible migraines to those of us who are more sensitive to these chemicals.

It is also incredibly taxing on our liver and kidneys to try to process these toxins from our bodies, causing many individuals to live with a higher risk of liver and kidney failure. Using the Kundalini lifestyle so that we exercise the proper diet and yoga regime will come a long way in helping us heal from these hindering effects so that we may live our lives to their full potential.

Water is also crucial in the cleansing of our human forms. Human beings are essentially created of water and therefore ingesting a healthy amount of water each day will help us clear every channel that runs through our bodies. Water flows quite similarly to the way the energy flows through our Nadi. Using water in our meditational exercises to add sound and visual strength to our practices is always a wise decision, but making sure we are frequently ingesting water to rehydrate fully is essential.

Ingesting the proper nutrients that we need through the form of juicing is an excellent way to promote our bodies to heal and rid itself of any toxins. Many different programs available offer a wide variety of helpful fruit and vegetable juice recipes that will help us detox our pineal gland as well. The power of the earth once again stands out substantially in the many useful tools that are provided to us to encourage healing. It is a wise decision to try adding juicing routines to our Kundalini lifestyle so that we can help boost the strengths in our bodies that are needed to rid us of toxins and help loosen the blocks in our Nadi.

Juicing diets are a reliable approach to healing and must not be treated as such to avoid overloads in our detoxification. It is entirely possible for individuals to experience a type of "healing crisis" while undergoing strict juicing and exercise regimes. These crises are often brought about by our bodies going into a state of shock from the severe healing it is currently undergoing. Reports of the symptoms of a healing crisis are usually of flu-like tendencies with excess sweating, mainly from the hands and feet. This crisis is all because our bodies are putting their full energy into fighting and detoxifying whatever ailments is that are influencing us.

Our bodies will try to rid itself of all toxins through in any way it can during these crises, and horrible sweat waves are the most common and one of the fastest ways for our bodies to expel these ailments. Healing crises can sometimes lead to excess urination and even vomiting.

The fact of healing crises should never deter those from attempting ways to bring about natural detoxification, as they usually are strictly related to pushing ourselves beyond our limit and trying to speed up the healing process. If we take in too much of the powerful tools that detox and clear our blocks, our bodies will need to react just as fast and just as potently. Thus, if we make sure to monitor our practices and diets so that they gradually introduced into our lives, we can avoid situations that might prove more difficult for us to heal.

Activated charcoal is an excellent supplement that will absorb any toxins that reside within our circulatory system. Taking this supplement in the form of pills or even using the power with water to create a detoxifying paste is usually guaranteed to perform with excellent results. Activated charcoal is a frequent ingredient in many favorite beauty products today, especially common in facemasks and bath soaks. These detoxifying properties will help cleanse our skin as well, providing ease to ailments ranging from acne to bee stings or spider bites.

For those of us who struggle with muscle and joint pain, Kundalini exercises will strengthen our mind and bodies, but sometimes these pangs of discomfort can grow stronger after our practice. The use of Arnica gel combined with peppermint oil is an excellent determent to the aches in our bodies. After our Kundalini yoga exercises, using arnica and peppermint on our usual, or even new, sore muscles and joints will significantly lower their pain level.

Chapter 12 Elevate a higher state of consciousness with kundalini

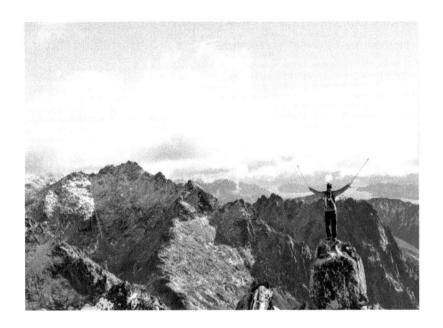

Have you ever had a feeling about something and you just know what others might not feel, or see? Have you ever heard the thoughts of another, but second-guessed that you did? Have you had a dream before that come true days later? Do you ever feel the presence of things that are not of the earthly realm? This is just scratching the surface of some of the things that begin to happen when you awaken your psychic awareness.

As part of Kundalini rising and the process of clearing and releasing blockages and negativity from your subtle body, you shift your perception of reality to the extent that you are able to crack open your latent abilities to receive input from other dimensions. This ability is not reserved for a select few or passed down genetically through generations, although that has been known to happen. This power to feel beyond the physical realm exists in us all and can be nurtured and grown into everyday use and understanding.

Many people have fear about this level of input because it can feel uncomfortable or vulnerable to tap into the unknown, into things that on the Earth plane we call magic, witchcraft, or superstition. Really, it is truly available to anyone to use this ability. When we are locked in our sleeping state (pre-kundalini rising), we cannot fathom the possibilities of such an existence, but as we allow our awakening to progress fully and reach the state of higher consciousness, we can open the brow and crown chakras to receive and accept our abilities as psychics.

These abilities can manifest in a variety of ways and have been reported as some of the side effects of the awakening process.

The next few subchapters will go into greater detail about the different kinds of psychic abilities that can be awakened, as well as techniques for opening and expanding these abilities.

Types of Psychic Awareness — The Clairs and More

Kundalini Awakening is all energy and when you begin clearing all the blocks and wounds, negative vibrations and old programming, you rebalance your true energy and become a clear channel of energetic flow. In the language of psychic capabilities, having clearness relates directly to each of the many forms of psychic understanding. You have to be clear (Clair) to work with these powers.

Once you have opened your Kundalini energy and you begin to experience the impact and effects of clearing your energy field, your latent psychic abilities can start to surface and may manifest in one, some, or all of the following ways:

- Clairsentience - This psychic ability simply means 'clear sense'. It is a knowing, or sudden understanding of emotion, or physical feelings from someone outside of yourself. It can also be a place like a building, a shop, someone's house, and you get a feeling about it and just know that it is comfortable, or unsafe, or has a negative history, or something bad happened there. This is sensing what is not seen but is very present.

- Clairaudience - Audience refers to audio and audio refers to sound. The clear hearing or clairaudience describes the ability to channel energy in the form of hearing tones, music, words, thoughts, and information from spiritual guidance, angels, and even loved ones who have crossed over.

- Claircognizance - Cognizance is the term relating to knowledge and awareness. Clear knowing is similar to clairsentience, except that claircognizance is knowing some form of knowledge without studying it or being told by another. It is knowing of information, while clear sensing has more to do with feelings.

- Clairvoyance - This sense involves the ability to clearly 'see', which often occurs in the form of inner visions through the mind's eye, or the ability to perceive auras of people, objects, animals, etc. This can also relate to clearly seeing the energy of spiritual entities, or spirit guides, but this visioning can also occur, again, in the mind's eye. The images seen in the third eye chakra can appear as clearly as a photograph or a movie.

- Clairscentist - This sense pertains to an ability to clearly smell scents from a spiritual distance. It may mean picking up on smells such as tobacco, lemon zest, or roses, because of their association with people close to you in your life, or who have crossed over and are sending you a message. It could merely be a sense of people you are about to come in contact to or a collection of energies.

- Clairgustant- The sense of taste can be connected to your psychic sense, allowing you to taste something not of your own sense of taste, nothing you ate or drank, but someone else's. This could happen if you are doing an intuitive reading for someone, or you are at a cocktail party and you know what the person you just met had from the hors-d'oeuvre tray.

- Clairtangency - This sense describes a clear touch. For people with this sense, they can pick up an object and know its history, where it was made, whether it was well cared for, who owned it, etc., or they can just get a positive, or negative sense about the object.

It also works with touching another person. For example, laying a caring hand on the shoulder of a person you are offering compassion to and feeling all of their emotions, fears, sorrows, and so forth. Another word used to describe this ability is psychometry.

- Clairempathy - This sense allows for the ability to clearly understand emotions. This is sometimes considered a form of telepathic communication, as though you can tap into the brain wave energy of someone's emotional experience. It can relate to animals and places, as well as humans and is a direct understanding of your own emotional state and from there, a sense of another's internal attitude or emotion.

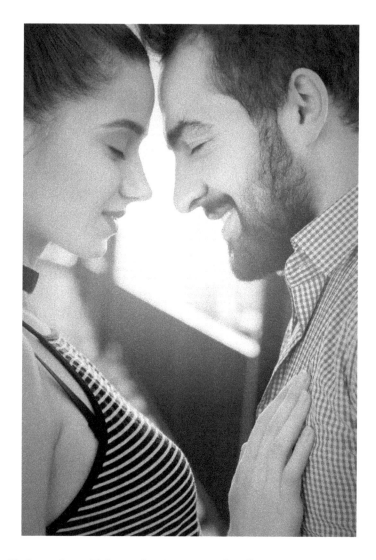

- Telepathy - Telepathy is scientifically proven to exist not only in humans but animals as well. When you are vibrating at a high frequency and your channels are clear, you can connect to another through brain waves which go from Beta (consciousness and reasoning), through Alpha (deep relaxed states), to Theta (light sleep/meditation) and finally on to Delta (deep sleep). Another brain wave measurement, Gamma, is the 'insight' brain wave that allows for eureka moments, and enlightened consciousness.

- In telepathy, you can fall into rhythm with another person's brain wave patterns and communicate thoughts, feelings, ideas, and images. This is easier in an alpha or theta state so that your logical mind (beta) won't reject the concept.

- Projection - The practice, or ability to project one's energetic body (astral/subtle) into other places, realities, or dimensions. It can be just a sense of these places, or experiences, though some have reported what feels akin to an 'out of body' experience (which makes perfect sense if your subtle body leaves your physical body to go on a trip). This travel, or projected experience, can also occur in the third eye and can be associated with clairvoyance, where you visit these inner realms in that chakra.

- Precognition - This is the ability to 'see into the future', essentially. Often, people with this power will have premonitory dreams that manifest in reality later. For the developing precognitive, it is important to study the symbolism of dreams and to not take them literally, but as messages of the higher self or angelic realms in the form of archetypal and symbolic imagery where your brain can understand and process. It can also manifest as an ability to just feel or know that an event, or situation is about to take place. For example, having a feeling that a guest is about to arrive and knock on your door, without any previous knowledge.

As you begin to develop your psychic senses through your awakening, you will discover that there are unlimited possibilities for how they can show up in your life based on your unique personality, characteristics, and background. Do not feel discouraged if this part of your awakening takes longer to know. It is important that if you are interested in working with your latent psychic capabilities that your intentions using these powers are for good and nothing else. Desiring psychic awareness to manipulate others, create disempowered feelings in other souls, or to serve only the self, will create negative energy blocks in your chakras which may prevent your ability to work well with this ability and hinder your awakening journey. The more you know about all of the above capabilities and how to nurture them, the clearer your knowing of enlightenment and oneness with the whole universe.

Developing Your Psychic Capabilities

Finding the appropriate lessons to exercise your psychic awareness can be challenging. There is plenty of misinformation on the world wide web, and sometimes the resources found in books are hard to find. There are, however, the right sources of information and it is up to you to follow the trail of breadcrumbs.

Step 1: Let the Information Come to You

I realize the idea of waiting for the information you need to find you sound a bit wacky, and if you are feeling any impatience to get started, untimely. Often, when we are opening our psychic awareness, it involves working with the energies of the Universe to be a guide to the right source. Has someone ever given you a book out of the blue and said they thought you just needed to have it? Have you been looking for something and it shows up out of nowhere in your email or conversations?

When you are on the awakened path and you are cultivating your psychic awareness, it is important to allow the information to come to you. The Universe knows what you are searching for, and indeed, what you are ready for next on your journey. So just practice openness so you can be aware when these things pop up. Your intuition will confirm you are on the right track. Trust it.

Another way this can manifest is in the way of claircognizance, clairsentience, and clairaudience. Pay attention to the message you are receiving from other realms, dreams, and your own intuition and inner knowing. Your psychic abilities will develop in tandem with you looking for ways to practice them.

Step 2: Clair-Anything Means Clear Energy
If you are going to work on nurturing your emerging psychic senses, it is important that you remain energetically clear so that you do not misread or misinterpret messages, or emotions. Throughout this book, there have been several levels of energy clearing methods and techniques, without which Kundalini awakening and enlightenment would not be possible. Energy is key. If your channels are blocked from your own, or other people's negative vibrations, you will have a harder time giving and receiving psychically.

Developing an energy clearing ritual for everyday use can be very beneficial. This could be as simple as using sage, or incense to smudge or cleanse your home and body after several people have been around you and brought their own negative vibrations into your space. This can energetically disrupt your ability to clearly 'see'. Salty baths can be very helpful, as well as spending time alone in nature to recharge and ground your energy.

You can do these things before you engage with any exercises to develop your psychic awareness, or just in general, to keep your vibration elevated for your awakening process. Incorporate some of the yoga postures and breathing exercises to help keep your channels clear too.

Step 3: Trust Your Own Knowing
It seems like magic, to go from being unawakened and in no way psychic, to being enlightened, full of love and light and able to tap into the energies of all existence through clairsentience and other means. When these things start opening up inside of you and manifesting in your reality, since you have never felt it before, it might feel odd, uncomfortable, or scary. Many people can be ostracized by our society and called crazy or schizophrenic because they can hear, or see what no one else can. Imagine if those abilities were nurtured instead of medicated and cut off.

No one will have a Kundalini awakening experience quite like yours. The journey will bring you closer to humanity and the whole Universe, but it will be your soul's road to travel. Self-trust is invaluable along this path. Your quest as an awakened soul is to know and trust your divine truth and honor your creative power.

Opening your psychic sense or sixth sense as it is often called demands your trust. Trust your visions and projections. They are your reality. Trust your sense of something. Trust your connection to otherworldly beings and energies. They are here to help you and offer guidance. Do not ignore it when you hear it, see it, sense it, feel it, know it. That is your gift and it is yours to share with the good intention of all.

A word of caution on opening these abilities into your life: check your ego at the gate. This is nothing to brag about. Anyone can do this, especially when they release their Kundalini energy and experience awakening. There is little room for big heads in using your psychic light. You need to have plenty of space in that head to help others in need.

Step 4: Collaborate with the Cosmos

Enlightenment is free. Transcendence is for everyone. It crosses time and space and all realities. There is not a person alive on this Earth who does not share your ability to know this truth. Awakening comes to all those who seek it and answer its call. Connecting to the other realms of life, forces of nature and cosmic beings is an answer to your soul's desire to know all.

Believe you are known by all that is, by the Universe. Ask to know and you shall receive knowledge. Speak to your knowledge, speak to your energy, tap into your light and primal force. It is always talking and when you speak, listen, and then you will hear the answer.

Chapter 13 Increase Psychic Intuition and Mind Power

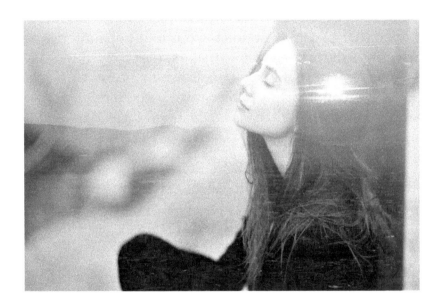

M any people are familiar with what the intuition is, but what exactly is the intuition? Some people say that it is the highest form of intelligence. Intuition is the ability to know something without evidence or analysis. It is about knowing. Sometimes, when the phone rings, you simply know who is calling.

The truth is that the intuition is very common. Unfortunately, today, people do not recognize it. Many people do not take notice of the messages from their intuition and only rely on logic or the use of reasons. Hence, they fail to listen to what the intuition tells them. Once they get used to shutting down their intuition, then they reach the point where they can no longer hear or notice it. The good news is that it is never too late to learn to listen to your intuition again.

How to develop your intuition

The best way to develop the intuition is simply by using it. If you have not paid attention to your intuition for too long, then now is the time for you to make some changes and start listening to your intuition again. Learn to listen to how you feel. A good approach is to recognize your emotion or "gut feeling" and then use reasons to justify it instead of relying on reasons alone.

It is also worth noting that the practice of meditation is a natural and effective way to develop the intuition. All the meditation techniques in this book will develop your intuition. Here is another interesting exercise that can enhance your intuition:

Use your intuition in your daily life. For example, when the phone rings, try to "guess" who is calling. When you are at the supermarket or when driving, visualize the first person whom you will see before you take a turn. There are many other ways to put your intuition into work. The important thing is to make use of it regularly. Do not be discouraged if you commit mistakes. The more times that you use your intuition, the more you will get good at it.

How to Develop Your Psychic Abilities

Enhance your psychic abilities.

We have already discussed notable psychic abilities that you can learn. Now, how do you enhance these abilities? Well, just like with any other skill, you simply have to keep on practicing them. When you say practice, it means actually putting it into real application. The best way to practice is to incorporate your psychic abilities in your everyday life.

So, how do you live with psychic abilities? Simply make them a natural part of who you are as a person. After all, there is no good reason for you to hide them. However, it should be noted that you should not boast about your abilities, and you should not use them for evil purposes. Let us now discuss effective ways on how to enhance your psychic abilities by making them a part of your everyday life:

When you take a bath, do not just clean your physical body, but also make an effort to cleanse all negative energies of your astral body. Visualize that as you clean your physical body, you also clean all negativities and impurities in your soul. See and feel the negative energies being washed away by the water and go in down the drain. Visualize yourself shining brightly.

If you have time to focus on your breath, then you can cleanse and charge yourself at any time. As you inhale, visualize positive energy entering your body. When you exhale, see and feel the negative energies being released from your body.

When someone calls you on the phone, take a moment to define who it is. Close your eyes or just focus, listen to your intuition, and then focus on who it is.

When you are engaged in a conversation, do not just listen to the words that the other person is telling you. You should also connect to them on a deeper level by using your empathic ability. Use whatever technique you may find helpful or necessary.

Make sure to make time to meditate regularly (every day). Meditation plays a very important role in your spiritual development, especially in the awakening of the Kundalini.

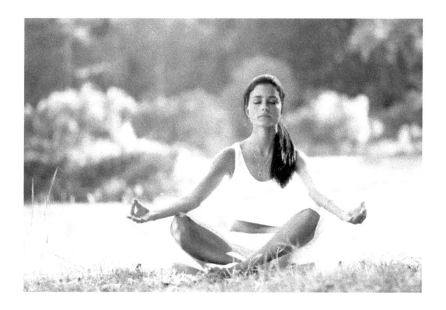

When you see an interesting object, especially if it is an old object, hold it in your hand, feel it, and allow your intuition to tell you the history of the object. This ability is known as psychometry.

Start using your intuition. This does not mean that you should no longer use logic or reasons, but you should also pay attention to what your intuition tells you.

Improve yourself by working on corresponding chakras.
There are many ways to incorporate your practices in your daily life. The problem is that there are people who simply do not take the efforts to practice their abilities. It is also advised that you give yourself even just an hour from time

to time to do nothing but to practice your abilities. You do not have to develop all your psychic abilities all at once. If you want, you can just focus on one or two abilities at a time.

The more that you make good use of your abilities, the more that you can develop them. The key here is repetition. This is why continuous practice is very important. You also have to give it your focus and attention. Always do your best.

Use Your Mind's Power to Heal from Within

Your mind is one of your most powerful assets. However, most people do not know where to begin when it comes to harnessing it. The good news is that harnessing the depths of your mind and their power is not hard. It is all about knowing which strategies are most effective and how to use them.

You want to start by expanding your awareness. This will make it much easier for both information and energy to start flowing through your mind. You will have a lesser vulnerability to toxic and negative emotions and it will be much easier to process information and take advantage of the energy inside you. Bad habits that you want to break, such as smoking cigarettes or overeating, are much easier to tackle when you are using the full power of your mind and have a high level of awareness. You will also enjoy much greater balance, flexibility and creativity.

There are several things you can do with your mind to take full advantage of its power, including:

Those who expect treatments to work, such as for a medical condition, may help to make the treatment more effective. In fact, a study was performed that showed that pain relievers for general headaches work better and faster when the person taking them believes they will work better and faster.

Know your purpose in life and focus on it to live longer. If you wake up every day knowing what you want and need to do, you help to increase your longevity.

Use a gratitude journal to improve sleep. One of the biggest causes of insomnia is focusing on the negative before bed. A gratitude journal puts you in a positive frame of mind, allowing you to sleep better.

Get sick less often, when you are optimistic since this has the potential to naturally boost your immunity. Research shows that the people who tend to get sick the least also tend to be among the most optimistic.

Imagine or visualize working out to build must. This might sound strange, but some studies have been done looking at this. One showed that a 24 percent increase in strength was achieved by those who simply worked out via visualization.

Use meditation to slow the aging process. This is no surprise since stress ages you and meditation works to alleviate stress.

Make sure to laugh loud and often to decrease the risk of heart disease. When you laugh, stress hormones are decreasing, according to multiple studies.

Research shows laughing can also decrease artery inflammation and improve your good cholesterol.

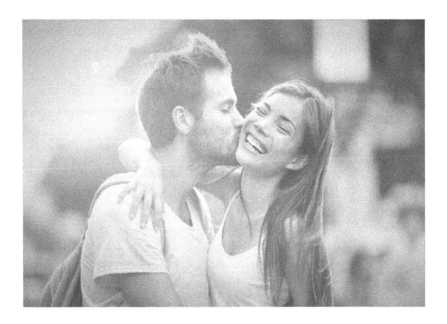

You can see that the mind can positively impact all areas of your health and life when you know how to use it. Now that you know the potential, it is time to start harnessing it. The following help to make this possible:

- Keep an open mind at all times
- Be clear about your life's passions and have passion for everything
- Avoid rigid beliefs, judgment, prejudice and anything else that can close down an open feedback loop
- Make sure that you always consider other points of view
- For conscious choices, always taking responsibility
- Never use denial for incoming data to censor it

- Look at guilt, shame and other psychological blocks, identify them and find ways to block their control over your thoughts and mind
- Make sure that you are truly emotionally free
- Spend time every day being willing to redefine your values, thoughts and your total being
- Never keep secrets
- Let the past go, learn from it and never regret it
- Never be fearful of the future, but instead embrace the possibilities

Breathing and be aware of it is an important element concerning being mindful. Find a place where you can sit comfortably that is quiet and free from distractions. Close your eyes and focus on your breathing. Listen to the gentle sound that happens when you exhale. Open your eyes and watch as your chest rises and falls with every breath. Remember the mantra, "breathe in, breathe out" and you go through the process. Try to clear your mind of everything except the focus on your breathing.

Conclusion

Thank you for making it through to the end of Kundalini Awakening, I hope it was informative and provided the information you needed to achieve higher spiritual awakening, peace of mind, healing, understanding, and the knowledge necessary to begin you down your magnificent path of Divine healing. No matter where you are in your journey of awakening, I hope that you achieve true happiness and peace of both mind and soul.

I also hope that Kundalini Awakening will encourage readers to reach out to others and help build a better community by applying the teachings of the Kundalini lifestyle in our daily lives. May the light you bring to others shine bright and strengthen the flame of those who burn weakest. If we follow the guidance of our Kundalini and trust our spiritual judgment, the awakening of the third eye and exploration of the Fifth Plane will become an easy achievement. Now that you have learned the magnificent power of manifestation and the positive effects it can have on our lives, I hope that you will continue to enhance your spiritual ability and continue your journey into the magnificent world of Kundalini health and awakening.

The next step is to apply everything that you have learned and start developing your psychic abilities and awakening the Kundalini. Continuing forward through ascension starts with creating the practices outlined in the book. Seek out yoga practices and meditations that will keep your creation consciousness flowing. Practice breathing exercises whenever you can. Continue to

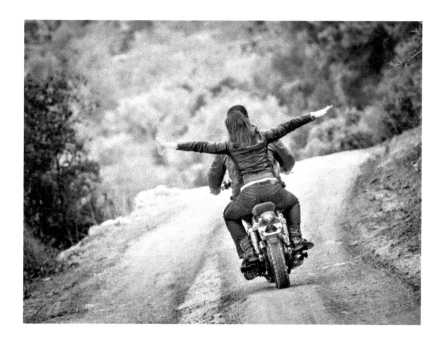

evolve and transform your alignment and chakra balancing. If you have already begun your Kundalini awakening experience, I guarantee you are not alone.

There are people everywhere exploring this journey. It is up to you to go forward on the path to finding the power of the divine within you. The journey is not always easy, but it is worth it. This is just the beginning and there is so much to uncover along the way. Now that you have gained some knowledge about the practices and effects of kundalini awakening, I hope that you are ready to commit to your journey so that you can live awakened, opened, and enlightened.

KUNDALINI MEDITATION

MORNING MEDITATION FOR BEGINNERS. HOW TO MAKE YOUR DAY MAGIC WITH KUNDALINI AND HOW TO INCREASE ABILITIES AND EVOLVE YOUR SPIRIT. FEEL AMAZING EVERY DAY AND NO ANXIETY WITH YOGA, AND MUSIC

Introduction

This book is meant to be a guide written by a person just like you, who has learned about Kundalini through personal practice. The words within these pages are not being compromised by some hidden agenda. You do not have to be a follower of a specific tradition. All that is required is that you have a mind and heart that are open to receiving wisdom and love.

You will find practical useful information and not some theory that you cannot interpret. The world is full of complex practices, so we will be looking more at the straightforward information.

I will share with you the different areas of Kundalini awakening and the journey you will take. Everything in this book, whether explicitly Kundalini or not, will help you to reach the enlightenment that you desire.

With this book, you can reach your enlightened purpose in life. Your life will have new meaning. This is a long journey, but it is one that you will enjoy every step of the way.

Chapter 1 What Is the Kundalini? And Why Is It So Important to Learn Kundalini?

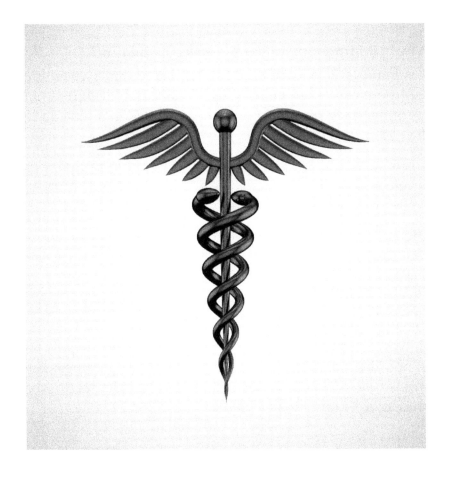

What is Kundalini?

The Kundalini, also known as goddess power or serpent power, is said to possess immense power. It is located at the base of the spine. The practice of awakening the Kundalini is very much known in India, but it is also being practiced in different parts of the world. The Kundalini is said to look like a coiled serpent at the base of the spine. Once awakened, it becomes a gateway or a key to great psychic powers, and even enlightenment.

Why is it important to learn/practice Kundalini?

It is important to learn and practice Kundalini awakening because it can take you to a higher spiritual level. It is not uncommon for people to suddenly be stuck in a plateau in their spiritual life.

It is a state where there seems to be no more progress or development. During this stage, awakening the Kundalini is often one of the best things to do.

Of course, you do not need to be in a spiritual plateau before you learn and practice to awaken the Kundalini. In fact, this is something that you can do at any time.

If you want to go deeper into spirituality, if you want to be able to harness psychic powers, then this is the one for you. However, it should be noted that acquiring psychic powers is not the primary goal of Kundalini awakening. The acquisition of such powers is merely incidental to the process of Kundalini awakening.

The differences between Kundalini and Prana

Some people confuse Kundalini and prana with each other. It should be noted that these two terms are related to each other, but they are not the same. Prana is the pervading energy that exists inside you and all around you. When the Kundalini is awakened, a strong rush of prana surges through the body. Take note that Kundalini and prana are different from each other.

However, in some sense, it can be said that Kundalini is also prana. This is because of the belief that literally everything is made of prana. However, technically speaking, they are not the same, just as a chakra is different from Prana.

The Kundalini is often awakened by drawing more prana into the location where the Kundalini resides, which is at the base of the spine. Clearly, they are not the same.

The relationship between Kundalini and Chi

Chi is another term for prana. Prana is referred to by different terms depending on the culture or location. In China, prana is called as chi. In Greece, it is referred to as pneuma. In ancient Polynesia, prana was called mana. The term prana is a term that is used in India. Still, all these terms refer to the same energy. As we have already discussed, it is obvious that chi is not the same as Kundalini, for reasons already stated.

The health benefits of Kundalini

The awakening of the Kundalini has been linked to various health benefits. It promotes good health at many levels. It regulates and corrects blood pressure; it is also an effective stress reliever; it can fight and even cure diabetes and other diseases, as well as a host of many other physical benefits.

This also involves relief from stomach and liver problems, even issues with kidney stones and gallstones. There are even those who claim that awakening the Kundalini can cure serious diseases like cancer. Indeed, when you experience the power that surges through your body upon awakening of the Kundalini, you will know that indeed, everything is possible. Having clarity of thought is a very common benefit of awakening the Kundalini, as well as increased focus, attention, and mental power.

It is also worth noting that many of these benefits can be enjoyed even without fully awakening your Kundalini. The different practices themselves, as you will learn from this book, can give you tons of health benefits. Of course, if you want to experience the benefits to their fullest potential, then you need to actually awaken your Kundalini.

Different Kundalini exercises and meditations

It should be noted that there is no single exercise or meditation technique that will guarantee the awakening of the Kundalini. The accumulative spiritual practices and spiritual maturity are needed for this to happen. All the practices in this book will help you awaken your Kundalini. However, be reminded that gaining knowledge is not enough. You also need to put that knowledge into actual and continuous practice.

You may wonder why this book is full of mental and meditative techniques. The reason is that the awakening the Kundalini is more of a mental effort and practice.

You should expect to engage in long hours of meditation. However, there are also physical exercises that can help you awaken the Kundalini.

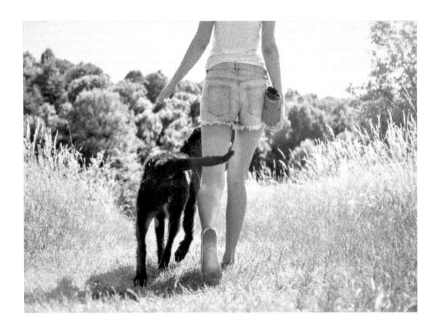

After all, physical exercises of any kind are a natural way of cleansing the body of negative energies. Depending on your physical fitness, you may engage in a physical activity or exercise of your choice. For starters, you might want to engage in some walking exercises.

If you are a feeling fit and healthy, then you can go for a jog or a good run. Needless to say, exercising is also good for the physical body.

The best way to awaken the Kundalini is by doing meditation. As you read this book, you will learn different meditation techniques. Some of these meditation techniques will directly empower and engage your Kundalini, while others may do so indirectly. Still, it is worth noting that all meditation practices help in awakening the Kundalini. Hence, you can rest for sure that no effort will ever be wasted.

The effects of Kundalini activation on the body, emotions, and the mind

As we have already discussed, awakening the Kundalini offers tons of benefits to the physical body. As to the emotions, it will make you feel more centered and calm. In fact, even before you reach the stage of awakening, you will already enjoy its positive effects on the emotional level. You will feel less stressed, and you will be more in control of yourself and your emotions.

With regard to the mind, you will have more mental clarity. You will be able to think and analyze things more clearly. It will give you such clarity that you have never experienced in your life. In fact, it is with such mental clarity that is tantamount to having complete peace of mind.

How Kundalini feels

If your Kundalini is still dormant, then you might not feel it at all. However, the more that you work on your Kundalini, the more that you can feel it, especially when you do the meditation techniques that directly engage the Kundalini. At the moment of the awakening of the Kundalini, you can expect for a powerful rush of energy through your body.

How to clear the blockages that prevent Kundalini from rising smoothly

Blockages can prevent the awakening and rising of the Kundalini. In order to avoid this from happening, you need to ensure that there is a free flow of energy through the energy channels meridians. You should also ensure that your chakras are cleansed and aligned.

However, what causes these blockages? There are many causes of blockages. A common cause of this is having too much stress. In the modern world, being stressed has become very common; and this is actually a sad thing, as it means that many people do not enjoy a free flow of energy. If you want to activate your Kundalini, then you need to be sure to manage your stress levels effectively. It should be noted that stress itself is not bad; it is when you fail to manage it properly that it becomes bad for you. There are many other causes that can impede the free flow of energy, such as having bad experiences, emotional breakdown, psychic attacks, and others. When treating blockages, it is important to note the reason or the main cause of the problem. A common mistake is to treat a blockage without attending to what causes it in the first place. Therefore, if a blockage is due to your stress at work, then you need to make some adjustments at work. You cannot just treat the effect or the result without going after the source.

Therefore, removing of any blockages or healing should be done on two levels, physical and spiritual. On the physical level, you may have to make some lifestyle changes. On the spiritual level, then you need to do the meditations as will be discussed in detail later in the book.

148

How to awaken a dormant Kundalini

As already mentioned, there is no single rule or practice that can guarantee the awakening of the Kundalini. This will have to depend on your overall spiritual

maturity and practices. However, generally, there are two ways to awaken a dormant Kundalini: by yourself or with the help of a spiritual master.

Being able to do it on your own is exactly what this book is about. However, if you want to do it with the help of a spiritual master or guru, then this would involve complete dedication and submission to your master. Your master may also require you to do certain meditation practices; however, there are also those who claim to be able to awaken one's Kundalini as long as the disciple relinquishes everything and submits to his/her master.

The problem here is that it is not easy to find a real master. Unfortunately, there are so many people out there who claim to be a master but are, in reality, just merely full of hacks and shams. Another problem with this approach is that although a master may be able to awaken your Kundalini, your soul might not be ready for it. This refers to your spiritual maturity. Therefore, when it comes to awakening the Kundalini, it is strongly advised that you do the work yourself so that your soul can mature and make you be ready for it. Of course, you are still free to ask help from a master but do not neglect your own spiritual growth.

Why is it important to learn/practice Kundalini?

It is important to learn and practice Kundalini awakening because it can take you to a higher spiritual level. It is not uncommon for people to suddenly be stuck in a plateau in their spiritual life. It is a state where there seems to be no more progress or development. During this stage, awakening the Kundalini is often one of the best things to do.

Of course, you do not need to be in a spiritual plateau before you learn and practice to awaken the Kundalini. In fact, this is something that you can do at any time. If you want to go deeper into spirituality, if you want to be able to harness psychic powers, then this is the one for you. However, it should be noted that acquiring psychic powers is not the primary goal of Kundalini awakening. The acquisition of such powers is merely incidental to the process of Kundalini awakening.

The differences between Kundalini and Prana

Some people confuse Kundalini and prana with each other. It should be noted that these two terms are related to each other, but they are not the same. Prana is the pervading energy that exists inside you and all around you. When the Kundalini is awakened, a strong rush of prana surges through the body. Take note that Kundalini and prana are different from each other.

However, in some sense, it can be said that Kundalini is also prana. This is because of the belief that literally everything is made of prana. However, technically speaking, they are not the same, just as a chakra is different from Prana.

The Kundalini is often awakened by drawing more prana into the location where the Kundalini resides, which is at the base of the spine. Clearly, they are not the same.

Chapter 2 Spiritual Growth

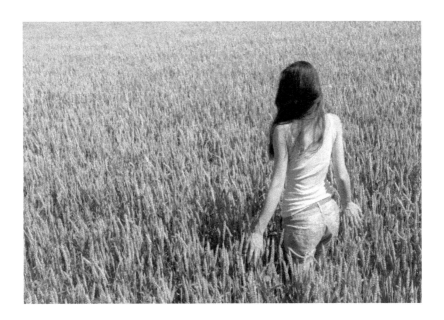

Kundalini awakenings happen differently for everyone. For some, they are slow and come in persistently but over time. For others, it can be extremely quick, almost like an explosion of energy in the gut area. Either way, Kundalini awakenings can be quite intense for anyone who experiences them. Here are some of the symptoms you can expect to experience during your awakening.

Remember, not everyone will experience all of the same symptoms. Even though the energy being awakened goes by the same name, recall the beginning of the book where we discussed that it is different from person to person, as each person is different. For that reason, you may or may not feel all of these symptoms in your awakening. Furthermore, you may experience some that have not been listed here. That is okay, too. The goal is to be one with the process and welcome anything that comes your way.

Everything Seems to Fall Apart

One of the first things many people experience in the face of their awakening is feelings of nervousness. As you awaken, it may feel like everything is falling apart. This is because the world as you have come to know it is being perceived through the eyes of someone who has Kundalini that is still dormant. As a result, you may feel like everything as you know it falls away.

Many people who awaken will experience massive life changes as a result of this falling apart. Several of the aspects of their lives that are not aligned with their awakened energies will begin to drift away as they make room for new, aligned experiences in their lives.

Although in the long run, this is generally all for the best, in the midst of everything falling apart you can feel intense bouts of chaos and stress. Sometimes, people will even block their awakening to lessen the chaos and prevent the stress from increasing.

Everything that has been used as a crutch to support your unhealed self will begin to render themselves as useless as you realize that they are no longer supporting you. This can, of course, be scary. Many call this "leaving their comfort zone" because they are venturing beyond the system they have carefully built around themselves to bring some peace and comfort into their lives. However, they will virtually always end up finding a more pure and true sense of comfort later in their lives when they enter a later phase of their awakening.

Physical Symptoms

Many individuals that undergo awakening experience physical symptoms as a part of the process. These symptoms are generally very random and are not linked to any health issues carried by the individual. Of course, if you do experience any ongoing physical symptoms that are particularly alarming, you should always contact your physician to rule out anything serious. However, realize that if nothing comes back and you remain "undiagnosed," it is likely that these are symptoms of your awakening.

Some of the physical symptoms people experience include anything from shaking to visual disturbances. Some will also struggle to relax as a result of the major rushes of energy that course through their bodies. Others still may even experience near-death experiences that either contributes to the awakening or are a result of the awakening.

Remember, whatever symptoms you experience, if you are at all concerned you should certainly contact a physician. Even though they may be spiritual awakening symptoms, it is always important to take proper precautionary methods and look after your physical body.

The reason why many people will experience physical symptoms is that their physical body is simply unable to handle such a rush of energy. As the awakening continues, these symptoms should subside.

The body will grow more accustomed to the incoming energies and will likely find it significantly easier to handle.

Feeling physical symptoms may encourage you to deny your awakening, but as long as you are truly healthy, enduring them can lead to powerful results.

If you are particularly concerned, you can always work alongside a Kundalini master to receive support and guidance in how to manage these symptoms and potentially slow them down to make them more manageable as you endure your awakening. In general, your physical, emotional, and energetic symptoms should last only about 20 minutes at a time.

Emotional Symptoms

Emotional symptoms are extremely common in Kundalini awakenings. In fact, they are felt by virtually everyone who experiences their awakening. Emotional symptoms vary, but early on the most common symptoms include ones like anxiety, despair, and depression.

The emotions can also range in the opposite direction, bringing intense feelings of elation, joy, and an overwhelming sense of peace to the individual.

These emotional fluctuations are directly the result of the changing energy within your body. At first, they may be intense and overwhelming. You may feel as though you are encountering and enduring many mood swings, which could make it challenging to deal with.

The best thing that you can do is allow yourself to embody the emotions and feel through them. Refrain from blocking them or resisting them, as this can result in you directly resisting your awakening.

Energetic Symptoms

The primary energetic symptoms experiences by individuals experiencing a Kundalini awakening are massive influxes of energies at seemingly random times. These energies can become quite powerful, resulting in people randomly feeling extremely energized and even restless. These energy symptoms are inevitable, as spiritual awakenings do exist in the non-physical life force energy of Kundalini. You may experience many symptoms as a result. Virtually all emotional and physical symptoms stem from the energetic symptoms of your awakening.

One interesting aspect of energetic symptoms is that many will go unnoticed. Because these are less tangible than physical and emotional symptoms, many things will actually go on in the background that will contribute to your overall shift. The best thing you can do to manage energetic symptoms is to find peace, allow them to flow, and work through anything that they bring your way either physically or energetically. The more you allow them to move through, the better it will become for you.

The Desire to Try Something New

After you have endured your chaotic episodes and the seemingly mass destruction of life as you know it, a new phase sets in. This phase includes feelings of curiosity and inquisitiveness. When you reach this part of your awakening, you will become more interested in trying new things. This is because all of the constructs you had built around yourself to protect your wounds are now fading and your wounds are being healed. Imagine it in a more literal sense: say you severely broke your leg. After several weeks of healing, your doctor says you are able to begin practicing walking again to rebuild strength in the leg. However, as a result of your fear, you decide that you are incapable of walking. You may even lie to the people around you to support this fear, constructing a safety net by having people expecting that you are unable to, rather than realizing that you are afraid of the healing process.

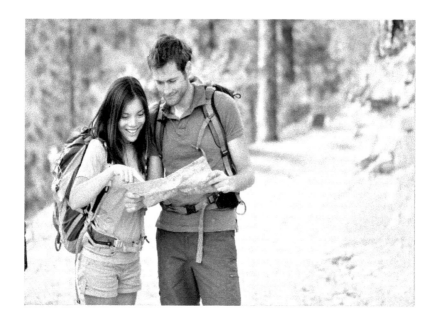

Now, imagine someone took away your means of transport, say perhaps a wheelchair or your crutches. As a result, you have to walk to accomplish anything. The safety and comfort construct you had built around yourself are now gone. At first, it is scary and chaotic. You are forced to face the truth. Eventually, however, you choose to face your healing, and you are able to walk again. With your newfound ability to walk once more, you might become curious about what else you can do. Can you run? Bike? Swim? You would likely begin exploring your renewed abilities to see how much you can really enjoy having two working legs.

The same goes for your awakening. Once you have healed from the false constructs you have built around yourself, you will want to explore. What exists when you are no longer protecting your wounds? You may begin traveling like you always wanted to. Or, you may take up new creative hobbies, make new friends, or otherwise explore the world around you. With your newfound ability to venture beyond your wounds, a whole new world of opportunities opens to you. Suddenly, you will want to explore and experience them all.

Miracles and Synchronicities Increase

Once you are actually willing to venture out and try all of those new things, another surprising symptom arises. Suddenly, you are receiving more miracles and witnessing more synchronicities than ever before. Support comes in from unexpected sources, and things will seemingly just "fall into place" for you. Your energies are aligned, and you are putting yourself out there, and now the energies of the world around you are meeting you at your new vibration.

Even more, healing happens. Only, now because you have experienced some of the hardest healing you will face in your awakening, you are curious. You have seen what healing can bring you, and now healing does not seem so hard and daunting. You are no longer available to hold space for you hiding behind false constructs of pretend comfort. You are ready to start healing almost immediately, realizing that on the other side of healing is where curiosity lies. Knowing that surrendering to the process of healing itself is a peaceful practice. Your perception changes, and as a result more comes into your life. More miracles, more synchronicities, more manifestations of the peace and joy you carry in your heart and soul.

Sensitivity Increases

We have already discussed how much your senses will be increased by your Kundalini awakening. So, instead of going into detail once more about how everything will awaken, I want to take you on a sensual journey for a moment.

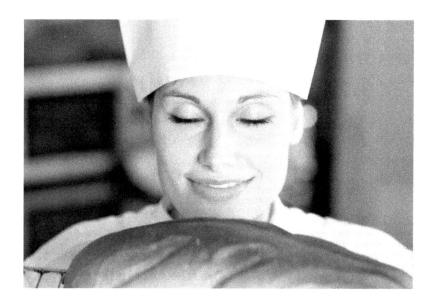

Self-Awareness Expands

One symptom that comes through your awakening is your expanding self-awareness. As you awaken, you will begin to realize things about yourself that you may have never noticed or taken the time to recognize before. You become aware of your internal energies, your intuition, and your inner truth.

Suddenly, you recognize patterns that no longer serve you. In fact, this very awareness is often responsible for the breaking down of your comfort zone so that you can experience true comfort in your life. You realize how you are feeling, the energies residing within you, and what you need to do to balance and manage these energies.

Your intuition seems to speak louder, and maybe you will become able to hear it for the first time. You will realize that your inner voice is, in fact, extremely powerful and has the capacity to serve you greatly in life. As you listen more, you begin to actually follow it. Suddenly, even more miracles and synchronicities are arising in your life. You are growing in your ability to realize that you are being guided, and your confidence to follow that guidance grows as well.

Lastly, your inner truth becomes crystal clear to you. You find that you are no longer searching outside of yourself for the meaning of, well, anything. You are able to trust your intuition, and trust that your inner truth is, in fact, true. You are then able to follow this truth and integrate it as one of your most respected sets of morals and values in your life. It operates as your guidance system, ensuring that you live in consistent alignment with your truth. Whenever you are curious as to whether or not you are living in alignment, you simply drop into your intuition and allow yourself to become aware of what it has to say. Then, you courageously follow its guidance and your alignment.

Compassion and Service Expands

One inevitable side effect of awakening is your compassion for others and your need to step into service. The more we awaken, the more we feel called to serve others. We quickly realize that one of the most valuable experiences we can have in life is not to acquire more material possessions or status, but to share the wealth of knowledge, joy, love, and otherwise with the world around us. We no longer feel confident in our ability to turn our eyes away from the tragedies being experienced by many on Earth. We find ourselves needing to become powerfully involved in the movements responsible for bringing peace, bliss, and equal opportunity to those across the globe. We want to end the suffering of others, not through shouldering their suffering, but through contributing to any means that we can. We share education, resources, materials, networks, and anything we can to compassionately bring healing to all who are ready.

You Develop a Sense of Purpose

Finally, one of the most fulfilling elements of the awakening process is that we integrate with our sense of purpose. We find ourselves understanding why we are here, what we are here to do, and what we need to do to fulfill that role. It becomes apparent to us where our unique energies are best spent, and we begin serving in that area. In many cases, our entire lives become devoted to service. We want to support everyone in every way that we can, serving tirelessly.

Most people will agree that when they are in service and fulfilling their sense of purpose in the world, they actually feel more energized. They are eager and excited to share, explore, and experience all that is associated with fulfilling their purpose.

When you have a sense of purpose, you are no longer clouded by distractions or a lack of motivation. You receive clarity. You understand why you are here, and you are able to operate in alignment with your truth and purpose to construct the most fulfilling life available to you. You embody your purpose and serve in powerful ways. In fact, your purpose may weave itself into every aspect of your existence. You become eager to learn more, you embrace the journey of understanding, and you serve in every way that you can. Suddenly, the need to be materialistically fulfilled by status, credit, wealth, or things that you own melts away. Instead, you feel devoted to serving in alignment with your purpose and feel deeply satisfied each time that you do.

Chapter 3 Aligning and Strengthening Your Chakras with Kundalini

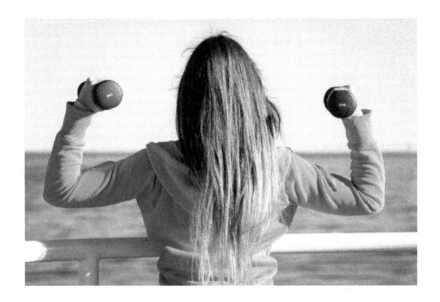

You learned a lot about chakras above, but there is still more information that you need. Having a deep understanding of chakras is imperative for making sure that yours are always in the best and proper alignment. The first step is learning about what can happen when your chakras are not in the proper alignment.

First Chakra

You might consider essential oils, such as clove, myrrh or cedar. Certain crystals can also be beneficial, such as bloodstone, garnet, smoky quartz, ruby, agate and hematite. The following methods are commonly used:

As much as possible, walk barefoot.

If finances are worrisome for you, set up a savings plan.

Around this chakra, engage in visualization where you see red flooding the chakra.

Each a variety of red food and spices.

Take the time to really dance.

Second Chakra

Essential oils for this chakra include ylang ylang and sandalwood. You might also consider working crystals into your healing strategy, including carnelian and moonstone. The following methods are commonly used:

Seek out and incorporate more orange foods and spices in your diet.

Take a relaxing bath with an array of candles and oils.

When you achieve something, make sure to take pride in it and celebrate.

Be kind and gentle with yourself.

Grab your favorite romantic movies and watch them often.

Around this chakra, engage in visualization where you see orange flooding the chakra.

Third Chakra

The essential oils you want to use include lemon and chamomile. You might also want to gather some crystals to help in healing this chakra, including amber, Tiger's eye and citrine. The following methods are commonly used:

Make time to get out in the sun and truly enjoy it.

Brew chamomile tea every day and enjoy it.

If you tend to talk badly about yourself, make sure to be aware of this and stop it before you get started.

Pack your diet that foods and spices that are yellow.

Make sure that the people in your life appreciate and love you.

Around this chakra, engage in visualization where you see yellow flooding the chakra.

Fourth Chakra

If you want to incorporate some essential oils into your healing strategy, consider bergamot and rose. In terms of crystals, the following are considered ideal for this healing this chakra: green jade, emerald and rose quartz. The following methods are commonly used:

Make sure that you do things that you love as often as possible. In fact, schedule time to do these things.

Identify your desires and dreams and do what it takes to follow them.

Be loving and generous.

Bring more green spices and foods into your diet. When you are talking to or listening to other people, make sure that you are always keeping an open heart.

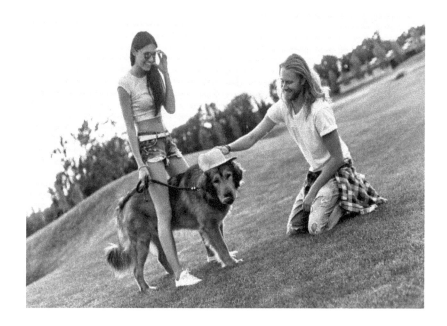

Around this chakra, engage in visualization where you see green flooding the chakra.

Fifth Chakra

The essential oils that can aid in the healing of this chakra include sage, lavender and neroli. When it comes to stones, you should incorporate aquamarine or turquoise into your healing strategy.

The following methods are commonly used:

Whenever you have the chance make sure that you sing.

Do not be shy about saying "no," but do so kindly.

With the people you have around you, make sure that you are honest and open.

If you find an authority figure that is hard to speak to, shine your love onto them.

Around this chakra, engage in visualization where you see blue flooding the chakra.

Sixth Chakra

There are a number of essential oils that are ideal for helping to heal this chakra, including jasmine, patchouli, rosemary, vetiver and basil. When it comes to crystals, you want to choose sodalite or lapis lazuli.

The following methods are commonly used:

When you are talking to someone, make sure that you listen closely to see if there

might be a hidden message.

If you use your intuition and get it right, make sure to give yourself praise.

Every person has their own energetic vibrations and you should world to feel this in

those around you and then try to determine if they are negative or positive.

Around this chakra, engage in visualization where you see indigo flooding the chakra.

Seventh Chakra

Olibanum and frankincense are the two essential oils that are the most useful for healing this chakra. Alexandrite and amethyst are the two crystals that you want to bring into your healing strategy. The following methods are commonly used:

Take the time to meditate.

In your daily routine, you should ensure that you get at least a little quiet time.

Incorporate foods that are purple, as well as grapes and blueberries.

Every day, read things that are inspirational and watch something that inspires you.

Around the chakra, engage in visualization where you see violet flooding the chakra.

Meditation Session 12: Compassion Meditation – 15 Minutes.

There are times when life gets tough and you may find yourself upset with a loved

one. This meditation session is focused on helping you to find your compassion to

forgive and let the negative feelings go.

Lie down on your back in a place you feel is comfortable, quiet and calming. Take a minute to push the negative thoughts from your mind. Close your eyes and start focusing on your breathing. Repeat the wishes you have for the person you are upset with. Wish them safety, happiness and health. After a few minutes, use the same wishes for yourself and repeat them. Imagine this person and you together enjoying each other's company. Remember that negative emotions only interrupt this relationship. As you come out of the meditation, gently stretch and leave the negative feelings you just released in the past.

Chapter 4 The origins of kundalini yoga and the journey of awakening your life-force

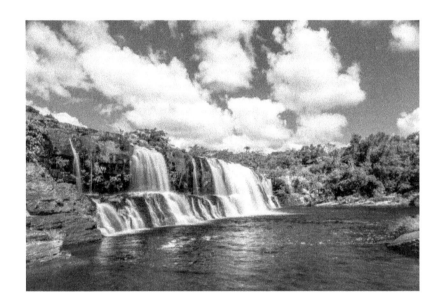

Though the exact origin of Kundalini Awakening is unknown, the sacred Vedic collection of writings, written between (c. 1,000 B.C. – 500 B.C.), is the earliest known material that mentioned it. This writing is known as the Upanishads. It is recorded that before Kundalini awakening was developed as a physical practice, it has already been known as a science of energy and spiritual philosophy.

Then this science of energy and spiritual philosophy was taught by masters to their students. With time, Kundalini Awakening was developed as a physical expression of the Upanishads.

For thousands of years, the public was not privileged to access the teaching about the Kundalini because it was kept secret. The knowledge was only with the master and he passes it across only to a trusted disciple to preserve the knowledge. It was believed that the public was not prepared to receive such powerful knowledge. It was Yogi Bhajan who broke this rule and made the knowledge open to the public to access in 1968.

Kundalini has a long and fascinating history. It seems to be the oldest of all philosophy and spiritual practice available today. It is not like other ancient religious philosophy or spiritual practices that hold onto strict rules or dogmas. Its flexibility and natural process has made it possible to move from one generation to the other. Individuals in each generation have found personal meaning and fulfillment for thousands of years. Its objective is selfless, simple and decentralized; helping people to actualize their Higher Self.

The Principles of Kundalini Yoga

The principles on which Kundalini Yoga was built are ancient, but still very relevant in the human experience today. Again, this spiritual energy starts at the base of the spine, and the process of awakening refers to how this energy spreads from your spine to the crowd of your head with time and practice.

The metaphysical aspect of the practices describes Kundalini as an awakening snake, from which emits an energy, or chakra that takes refuge in 7 locations in the body as you grow. According to methodology, the chakra energy rises through your being in the same way that air fills your lungs then disperses oxygenated bloods throughout the vital organs of your body as you exhale.

The goal is to ascend beyond the first 6 chakras and to access the 7th through what has been called, the "golden cord". This cord, as legend has it, connects pineal and pituitary glands. The significance of this is that those glands in particular are said to have been responsible for awakening the conscious mind of a human being. And not just with Kundalini Yoga — these glands are the subject of enlightenment in many current as well as ancient teachings. To access them is to finally see yourself and the world as it is, rather than as you think or hope it could be. The golden cord, in this particular practice, is the key to your awakening.

Kundalini Yoga combines the old teachings of three other, more specific yoga related spiritual practices. Each yoga focuses on an aspect of the human experience, from devotion (Bhakti), to power (Shakti), and mental fortitude coupled with control (Raja). Each gives an avenue on which to pursue a high consciousness, and well as to help you exploit your creative potential. It is in this way that these practices are said to be a practical technology for the conscious mind.

In addition to harnessing the power currently resting within you, Kundalini Yoga is said to release the practicing individual from the debt of karma. If translated to western terms, being released from one's karmic debts is essentially the same as being forgiven for the mistakes that you made throughout your life. It ensures that your soul is peaceful, and that even once you physically pass on, your soul will continue to be content. It is a very interesting concept, and is yet another spiritual benefit of Kundalini Yoga.

The Health Benefits of Yoga

We've discussed the power that Kundalini Yoga has to revolutionize and break your spiritual down to a very practical, very applicable level. But what of the physical benefits? Surely, such a sacred practice has to have a positive effect on the body and the mind along with the spirit? The answer is that it definitely does, and they even outnumber the spiritual benefits!

There is a plethora of ways in which yoga benefits the body – too many to count, in fact. So, let's explore 15 different benefits of yoga in daily life.

1. Improves flexibility – This is one of the most fundamental benefits of yoga. You may not be able to touch your toes or bend all the way forward in your first class, but you will notice over time that your body begins to loosen up, and with that will come a decrease in muscle pain as well.

2. Builds strength – Yoga is the best way to build a healthy amount of strength while balancing it with flexibility. The strength of your muscles contributes greatly to your posture, how you walk, and how you power the daily physical tasks that you may have. Lifting weights builds muscle too, but that (more often than not) takes away from your flexibility.

3. Improves posture – People underestimate the weight of their heads! When you slouch, the amount of tension of your heavy had leaning beyond your spines center of gravity can have lasting effects. Yoga encourages and promotes healthy standing and sitting positions, so you will learn over time how to sit and stand properly which will increase the longevity of your back and neck especially.

4. Stops joint/cartilage breakdown – The body is more like a machine than anything else. Like most machines, it has to be well oiled and taken care of with great compassion. Your cartilage is a spongey substance that cushions the area between your bones within joints. Yoga takes you through full ranges of motion that will loosen those joints and promote proper maintenance of your cartilage. Without going through the motions, your cartilage will likely wear with age, and eventually will be scraped down until you are experiencing the trouble and pain of two bones rubbing together without any cartilage between them. Many elderly experience this, hence why they most so slowly. Yoga can solve this problem!

5. Spinal Protection – Spinal disks are the shock absorbers of your back, and require a healthy amount of movement to stay limber and effective. In yoga, there are many motions that involve light twisting and turning to ensure that your spine stays strong and supple through the years. Back problems affect millions of people, so it only makes sense to find a solution that can remove you from that statistic!

6. Promotes bone health – This is important for women especially! You have seen the commercials about the prescription pills that are supposed to combat osteoporosis. Well, this is a natural, much less rigorous way to prevent it. The stances and poses that you take in yoga help to strength the bones of your arms and legs especially, which is where osteoporosis likes to start. In addition to that, yoga as a whole helps to lower the amount of stress hormones produced in your body, which lowers the rate at which calcium is lost in your bones.

7. Blood flow goes up – Although yoga isn't the same as running or lifting weights, it actually is much more effective at evenly distributing oxygenated blood throughout your body. In fact, going through the motions in a session promote a higher blood flow to the areas of your body that may not always receive it as they should (hands and feet). A consistent practice will also lead to more oxygenated blood circulating healthily through your organs and tissues, and even can help with people who have had heart or kidney problems and don't get the appropriate amount of blood to certain areas of their bodies. In addition to that, this increased flow reduces your chances of unhealthy blood clots.

8. Assists immune/lymphatic system – Everything in yoga from the contraction and stretching of a muscle, to transitioning between poses allows a fluid within immune cells to break free and "drain", if you will. As it drains, your body will be able to fight off infection more readily. It also makes it so that cancerous cells are broken down faster, and also so that the toxic waste within these cells is disposed of more quickly.

9. Improves heart health – Regularly increasing your heart rate during exercise can lower your risk of heart disease as well as the chances of depression because of the endorphins released during exercise. Yoga isn't an aerobic exercise by default, but there are variations that can be done in order to simulate a situation where your cardiovascular fitness is challenged. And even for yoga that isn't ass vigorous, it still lowers your resting heart rate and improves your overall endurance.

10. Lowers blood pressure - If you have HBP (high blood pressure), you too can benefit from yoga. The constant movement combined with the cardiovascular challenge will regulate your blood pressure, and eventually will lead to an overall drop due to the consistent practice of raising and lowering it with different forms of exercise.

11. Regulates adrenal glands – Cortisol is a stress induced hormone that appears when in a time of crisis, embarrassment, etc. Yoga reduces the amount of that this hormone sticks around. Which it first becomes present, it is helpful and makes you more alert, and even boosts your immune system. The real trouble comes when the situation that caused the increase passes and the cortisol sticks around. An overabundance of cortisol has been related to depression, osteoporosis, HBP, and insulin resistance (which can lead to diabetes). It also has been said that a constantly uninhibited influx of cortisol can lead your body to a state of crisis, and in this state the body stores most things that you may eat or drink as fat for safety purposes. Nobody wants that!

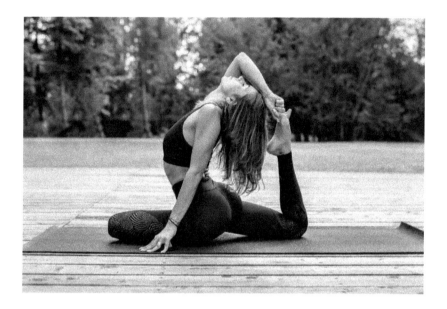

12. Improves moods – It is no secret that any form of exercise improves your overall moods, and promotes a happier existence. The consist practice of yoga will promote an increase in those "happy" hormones like serotonin and the endorphins that fill you with joy, which can be a great combatant of depression.

13. Encourages a healthy lifestyle – There is a spiritual, mental, and physical aspect of yoga. When combined, these things will trickle into other areas of your life from how to eat to how to you think act around others. Yoga encourages a heightened self-awareness, and in gaining a great appreciation for yourself, you will be more likely to begin taking better care of your wellbeing.

14. Fights diabetes – Yoga lowers your bad while increasing your good cholesterol. It makes your body more sensitive to insulin, while managing your cortisol and adrenaline levels which usually contribute to weight gain and the urge to take in more sugary foods. With a lowered blood sugar comes a lessened chance of attaining a heart disease, kidney issues, blindness, and other sugar-related diseases.

15. Improves focus – In yoga, there is no moment but the present one. The only way to master a pose is truly to focus within yourself, and to maintain that focus throughout your sessions. As your mind becomes accustomed to going to that present moment space, it will begin to show in other areas of your life as well, which can greatly improve things as small as driving to things as large as your professional career!

As you can clearly see, implementing yoga into your life would bring nothing but goodness into it. Now, imagine these health benefits coupled with what Kundalini Yoga can do for you.

Practicing Kundalini Yoga

The practice of meditation in Kundalini Yoga is designed to prepare the body for the surge of energy associated with the Kundalini Awakening. You are not yet ready for an awakening yet, and practice this yoga is what will prepare you. So, through Kundalini Yoga, you will learn how to ground your physical, mental, and spiritual self in order to allow for the energy within you to rise through your being. The focal point of many of these motions will be the base of the spine, the navel area, and other "anchors" of the body. These anchors, (or "stabilizers" in the exercise sciences) are the groups of muscles and bones that control your balance, posture, and overall flexibility. The breathing focuses on bringing the energy from those lower spaces to the highest center for your energy would exists at the top of your head as you exhale.

As a way to cleanse oneself too, there is another, more advanced practice of breathing in through one nostril and out through the other. The usual order is to breathe from the left to the right one. Kundalini Yoga is a tool for "psycho-spiritual" growth the maturation of the body, and each of these methods contributes to the larger picture of becoming an awakened individual.

Now, in order to fully awaken, there are 3 stages that you must progress through:

Stage 1 – This covers your first three chakras. During this stage, the primary objective is to clear yourself of all burdens. You see, the greatest inhibiting force preventing your energy from flowing freely is you. Injuries in the lower spine, unsavory memories, and negative emotions can all get in the way of your awakening. This ties back into how Kundalini Yoga assists you in erasing the karmic debts from your life experiences. The energy resting at the base of your being cannot come up until the path has been cleared to do so. In order to clear this path, you must be willing to face everything that ever brought you to your knees. This can be difficult for many people, because the truth can be a brutal and scary topic, but it must be done. Everything from the traumas of your past, to physical ailments, to the grudges that you've held, and even the control that you try to assert over your life—it all must be erased. And in regard to your physical challenge(s), it is more so the negative emotion attached to them that must be addressed.

This process will affect your physical, mental, a spiritual being in a heavy way. You will feel raw, and full of what may seem to be confusing emotions, but you will have to press on to continue to ascend. During this part of the process, you may also experience instances of feeling totally lost. This is a natural reaction because you are making such an impact shift in your beliefs that your subconscious mind will want to hold onto what you already know for security. But the trick here is actually to allow yourself to take the plunge.

You will know that you are making progress when you begin to experience true moments of peace, a sense of oneness with the world, and bliss. These feelings will be the direct result of opening yourself up, and getting rid of the unnecessary burdens and attachment to so much negativity that many of us hold onto in our lives. Your energy levels will randomly spike, as the impending second stage approaches. Whether you move forward though is up to you, because it will require that you continue to push the envelope of your mind.

Stage 2 – This stage is a very underrated one because many practitioners focus greatly on the first stage of a Kundalini Awakening, due to how much effort it takes to achieve. In the first stage, the physical and emotional obstacles are very multilayers, hence why so many time and energy is put into clearing those pathways. Once you are ready for the second phase of your ascension though, you begin to focus less on your personal experiences and more on a wider perspective of the world.

In this stage, societal, communal, and other broad categorizations will be the center of your attention. With this level of vision, you will begin to learn how to see yourself in others, and vice versa. In this understanding, you will see that emotions that were originally triggered by another person are actually just unhealed, or unresolved thoughts and emotions within yourself being shown to you through your interaction with that person. Sometimes, it can also be the other way around, or both! The point of it all though is to see life with a level of clarity that can aid you in getting the very best from your experiences.

In time, you will begin to see this in the entire world. The world will become your community, and each person in it a gift to your experience, because the ability to see oneself in others gives you the understanding to learn so much from those who pass in and out of your life. This is only the first half of the second stage though.

At the halfway point, this stage changes the lesson from how to clear yourself of your burdens, and more about how to gain the tools to attain your awakening. At this point, the original rawness of your emotions as well as your mental and physical state will die down. They will become replaced with more grounded and consistent feelings of peace and happiness. This period of time has been characterized as a time of "deep rest", but there still is much to do!

Now, you will begin to see how controlled life is on a wide scale, and hence will also begin to analyze as well as alter the way in which you once bought into societal patterns. We have all been conditioned from birth to act and think a certain way, so this step in the process exists to help you break free of that confinement. In addition to this, you also will relinquish your ego. By ego, I am referring to the letting go of idealism coupled with comparing yourself to others. No one but you are competition in this life, and you must cease in passing judgement unto others simply because they are different from who you are. You will learn that is okay to be different, and that judgement only comes from a place of arrogance.

During the first stage, there may have been a near death experience. Many of talked about having dreams about dying, or situations where they felt that threatened arising. It was not until the second stage that it all made sense though. It is at this stage in the process that even the thought of death becomes peaceful, and you learn to willingly accept all that comes your way. Therefore, you essentially go from a place of diving into the self, to seeing yourself as a part of a much larger picture, where all entities within hold significance.

Stage 3 – Stage 3 may actually be perceived to be the easiest of the three, but only because you have already laid the platform on which your ascension will occur. At this point, there no longer is the notion to "do", so much as it is an understanding that you must allow. The harder you try for something, the harder it will seem to attain. In truth, it (whatever it may be) is already yours—you just have to allow yourself to receive it by ceasing to control the things that are outside of your control.

This is the stage of contentment, where you will experience happiness, fulfillment, and a true love of self as well as others. No longer will you lean on the knowledge of others, because you now will understand that this journey is your own. The path of the awakened never ends, but once awakened, what happens from there will be up to you.

The energy that was once trapped within you can now flow outwardly freely, and will encapsulate your entire being.

The base from which the energy emits will become wider, and more receptive to you.

The actual time that it takes for this process to unfold really depends on the kind of person that you are. That has not to say there is any right or wrong kind of person to be — people just learn differently. So, no there is not any specific timeline. The goal is not to be do these things as fast as you can. The goal is to reach a place where you can literally change your life through practicing Kundalini Yoga. How long it takes shouldn't matter. The journey is the most important part here; not the destination. And in truth, there is no real destination! The process of learning is ongoing, and will stick with you through life and beyond death.

Chapter 5 How To Prepare Your Mind, Body, And Spirit For Kundalini Awakening

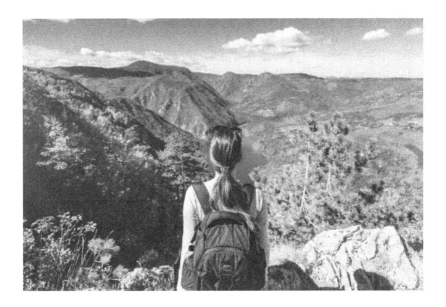

Now that you have a greater understanding of the chakras and the way Kundalini plays such an important part in the vibration and balancing of each chakra, you can now put some of these ideas into practice. If you are reading this book, no doubt you are curious about how to begin such a journey. Keep in mind, that this book gives a general overview of Kundalini energy and the process of awakening, but if you want to go deeper into the journey, don't hesitate to read more about it, take some yoga classes, and even connect with a Yogi or Guru, or a community of people who are on a similar journey, or who have experienced this awakening in their own life. I guarantee you, there are plenty of people out there, even in your own neighborhood, who are going through this process. We all have the power to awaken and having a community on such a journey can be not only helpful but also empowering. If you are not ready to take it to that level yet, just let this book be your guide as you unravel your understanding of these concepts.

Remember, awakening the Kundalini energy may be universal, but the experience will be unique to you, so stay positive and open-minded during the rising of your divine life-force.

There is not just one way your dormant energy becomes awakened. It can vary significantly from person to person. Some people practice yoga and meditation for years, working with Gurus before anything happens. For others, it can be completely spontaneous and caused by a buildup of traumatic situations, addictions or significant loss or grief, whether or not the person has any previous knowledge of what Kundalini even is.

There are plenty of stories like these which is why it is important to remain open-minded with yourself, but also all the other human souls looking for answers, or enlightenment.

If you decided to read this book, you have already begun this journey. Knowing more about it can help you feel more aware of what is potentially ahead for you, or even someone you know.

Preparing your mind, your body, and your spirit can be a great way to begin. Even if you have already experienced some of these things, this book can be a great resource to staying in balance or becoming more involved with the journey instead of letting it naturally unfold without any guidance or practice. Sometimes, when you let it unravel naturally, and don't practice any energy work, yoga, meditation or other balancing or healing practices, the experience can feel more chaotic and uncomfortable, more disorienting and unpredictable.

Finding ways to nurture yourself through awakening is key to a joyful and fully opening experience.

Each fundamental part of yourself can go through some preparations to allow for a more intentional awakening. Like you read before, for some people, it can happen spontaneously, but chances are, if you are reading this book, you are interested in and excited about starting that process of awakening your Kundalini and knowing your divine truth.

Below are a few, simple ways you can prepare your mind, body, and spirit to awaken.

Mind:

Daily affirmation.

Examples:

I am ready to align with my primal life-force.

I am one with the Universe and a part of All That Is.

I have divine energy within me and I am ready to wake it up.

I am open and accepting of everyone and everything.

You can always invent your own mantras to suit your needs better, but try to find ways to speak to yourself with the language and frequency of love. Say mantras first thing in the morning before work, while sitting in traffic, before bed, or any other time that feels appropriate.

Start practicing simple meditations, especially if you have never meditated before. Try not to overthink meditation. The point is to clear the mind of thought, but if the thoughts come, let them and then see them pass away from you like an ocean wave or a cloud. You can even find guided meditations online if you are not ready to guide yourself. Just search "guided meditation" and find what feels right for you.

Body:

Exercise. You don't need to join a gym or lift weights. You don't need to take aerobics classes or run 10 miles. Go for a walk around your neighborhood. Dance to a song you like in your living room.

Tread water in a swimming pool. Go for a hike on the trail. Just move your body in some way that feels pleasant, that doesn't feel like work, and that simply allows you time to get your blood flowing.

Stretch. You don't have to stretch every day, but a couple of times a week is very beneficial. You can practice yoga poses, or you can find a wide variety of places to find stretching routines, online, in books, or in a dance class at a studio.

One thing to keep in mind when you stretch: it is best to hold each stretch for a minute to a minute and a half. Your body needs the time to actually experience the result of the stretch. If you only do it for ten seconds, there won't be much of a change in your muscles and tissues.

Eat well. Diet has a great impact on the way we feel and our energy. As part of Kundalini awakening, you may have a natural inclination to change your diet, which has been commonly reported.

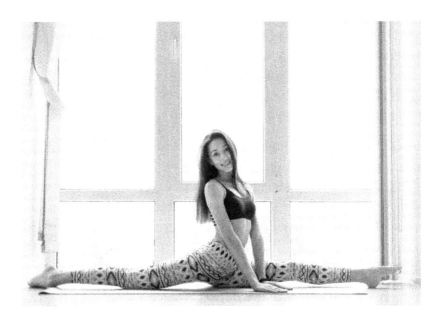

If you don't already, and to prepare for the experience ahead, start eating well by avoiding processed foods, alcohol, sugar and large quantities of caffeine.

Take it a step at a time if it's too much to do all at once. Eat more whole foods, vegetables, fruits, grains, lean meats, seeds. Drink a lot of water. Switch to tea instead of coffee.

All of this will start preparing your body for the adventure ahead.

Spirit:

Adopt a self-care practice. There are so many ways to do this. You can take a sunbath in the morning light and soak in the warmth and glow, focusing on your energy channels and how they feel as you relax. Draw a hot bath and add Epsom salt, preferred essential oils, and candlelight and spend quality time in the water letting your muscles soak. Lean up against your favorite tree with your favorite book and your favorite snack for as long as you want. These are a few examples to try or create your own ideas that resonate with who you are. The goal is to give yourself permission to love and care for yourself.

Keep a dream journal. The subconscious mind communicates so much to us when we sleep. In ascension, as the Kundalini rises, many people report having very profound dreams, premonitions, contact with spirit guides or astral travel experiences. Start keeping a dream journal to begin communicating with your dream world and your higher consciousness and look for messages from within.

Start a gratitude practice. It is proven that expressing gratitude, whether it be vocal, written down, or in the mind, can change your vibration frequency in a positive way. The concept of gratitude is a part of living as an enlightened human being. You can keep it simple. Begin by saying or writing things like, "I am grateful to have shelter and food to eat." "I have gratitude for the job I have right now." "I am thankful to be a part of this world." And so on. The great thing is, it can be about anyone and anything. The point is that thankfulness and appreciation is a valuable practice that brings you into closer alignment with your divine power and ultimate transcendence.

Start practicing these things today! It will be a helpful way for you to prepare for the quality of life you are looking for as you seek awakening.

Kundalini Sensations — How Does It Feel?

Kundalini Awakening is something you feel. You sense it with your whole being. These otherworldly and physical sensations, experiences, and visions are what draw people to seek answers to the intensity of awakening. Because it is not commonly discussed in our culture, or taught as a practice from an early time in life, when it happens it can feel rather shocking, especially when you aren't quite sure whether it is normal or not.

There is not a ton of information out there, apart from what you can learn in an ashram or from a guru. You can find some information across the internet and in books, but so much of this experience and practice isn't quite mainstream yet.

It is becoming more so as people are reporting more of their experiences through personal accounts on social media, in blogs, in yoga communities, or in their world travels.

It is the purpose of this book to expose some of the reality of why there can be hype revolving around these experiences, or why it is hard for some people to believe that this could really happen to all of us.

The Kundalini awakening process can take a long time since so many things need to shift, recalibrate, rewire, dissolve and eventually open for a transcended mind and wakefulness.

It is not an experience of immediate gratification.

If anything, awakening removes all need for instant gratification. It happens in many stages and manifests in many ways over a long period of time.

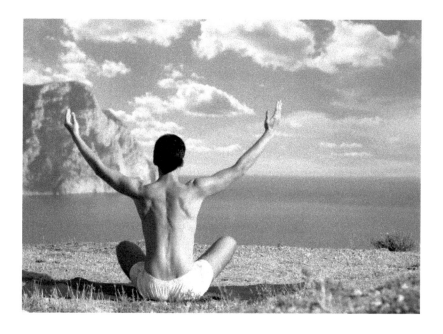

It can take years of experiences before you are truly awakened.

There are pre-awakening symptoms that occur and sometimes they ebb and flow for a while before you reach true divinity.

In the first phase of awakening, the dawning of your ascension, you may feel some or all of the following symptoms:

- Synchronicities with people, places, and experiences.
- Very vibrant, strange, and interesting dreams.
- Waking visions or lucid dreaming.
- Questioning the concept of God, religion, esoteric beliefs and agendas.
- Clearing and cleansing of ideas that resonate with old thought patterns and behaviors that are negative, inherited, outdated and/or against your truest self.

Intermittent nervous system reactions such as tingling sensations, itchiness or a feeling of something crawling in, or on your skin; uncontrolled muscle jerks, twitches or tremors; and electrical sensations moving within the body.

During the healing process associated with alignment and awakening, the body and mind can feel a variety of things, including some of the following:

- Headaches or migraines and pressure in the skull.
- Breathing changes.
- The tension in the muscles especially in the neck, back, and spine.
- Excessive heat, causing sweating, or excessive cold, causing shivering.
- Signs of emotional or mental health issues like anxiety, depression, and paranoia.
- A change in the thyroid that leads to an ability to sing well and in pitch (even if you have never sung before).

- Greater regularity and higher function in organ systems.
- Altered sleep patterns like insomnia or sleeping for excessive amounts of time, sometimes waking up really early in the morning, feeling well rested and enlivened.
- Restrained or declined sexual drive.
- Emotional highs and lows that are emerging as stifled and bottled emotions, or traumas from your past, present, or even former lives as a soul.
- The shift in body odor to more sweet and natural.

Some of these symptoms can derail your journey and you can stay locked in feelings of sickness, illness, or emotional trauma. It is important to remember that this is part of the ascension journey and that it will eventually subdue and subside. It is just your body and mind's way of healing and letting go of what no longer serves your divine, light energy. These symptoms can replay throughout the course of awakening.

Further along in the journey, after some of these initial feelings and sensations, there are experiences that have a more spiritual bent to them. You may feel some, or all of the following and also experiences not listed here:

A heightened sensory perception like an increased sense of taste, smell, seeing colors more brightly, sensitivity to bright light and loud or discordant sounds.

Intermittent nervous system reactions such as tingling sensations; itchiness or a feeling of something crawling in, or on, your skin; uncontrolled muscle jerks, twitches or tremors; electrical sensations moving within the body (continuing from earlier symptoms stages of awakening).

Increased understanding of the world rhythm and the dance of life; how we are all connected and a part of this primal, divine life-force.

Your crown chakra becomes open to receive "downloads" of information from the universe.

Flashes of light and energetic, electrical pulses in the body.

Having remembrances of past life experiences.

Meeting, or encountering spirit guides and otherworldly beings.

Beginning to understand your life or soul, purpose-why you are here.

Dissolution of illusions about your personality to reconnect with your higher self.

Unlocking of the pineal gland allowing for hearing internal, pleasant sounds inside the mind (*The pineal gland is also the source of our bioluminescence. It is the part of our body that biologically creates light*).

As your body continues to experience many of these symptoms, remember, these are just part of the process and the actual awakened state; the alignment with your divine essence is the ultimate goal.

As you become more awakened and more advanced in the journey, you will feel more of the following:

Descending into deep trances to the point of feeling like you have fallen asleep (this is where your energy really does a lot of clearing work, alignment and energetic downloads from the universe and higher consciousness occur).

Astral journeying and astral projection.

Change in diet (some people become vegetarian or vegan).

The decrease in and total lack of consuming substances like alcohol, caffeine, nicotine, and drugs.

Hormonal changes and rewiring of the brain to accommodate divine essence through thought and physical well-being.

Continuation of visions, otherworldly and mystical experiences, altered consciousness and connection with spirit guides.

Increase in sexual energy including spontaneous orgasms.

Unpredictable crying and/or laughter.

Euphoric and blissful feelings.

Detachment from acquiring worldly possessions like money or wealth, fame and glory, recognition for life's work.

Dissolving of the Ego.

The beginning phases and symptoms of Kundalini awakening tend to be the hardest part of the process. The reason is that we usually do not have any control over these experiences and it can be very confusing and uncomfortable.

The symptoms can be felt repetitively until all of the blocks, negative vibrations and former thought patterns and outdated beliefs are finally cleared to allow for true soul awakening. It is easy to lose focus of the end goal of alignment with your own benevolent nature and creation-energy, especially when it feels harrowing. That is why it is important to trust the process and let yourself dissolve into the awakening journey.

The possible sensations that can occur don't always happen exactly in that order. Because we all have unique life stories, personalities and karmic lessons to learn, your Kundalini awakening won't be exactly like anyone else's. That is another reason it can feel uncomfortable: it is your journey, your spiritual journey, your vision quest. It's beneficial to keep a journal of all of your symptoms, visions, phenomenal and mystical experiences so you can keep track of your journey.

Like with meditation, try not to overthink the symptoms. Know that they are all a part of clearing out your energy, your chakras, your mind, and your physical body to allow the Kundalini energy to rise and bring you into contact with your higher consciousness and spiritual alignment.

The Reasons We Meditate — Developing Meditation for Awakening

Meditation is not a new thing. It has been around in Eastern cultures and philosophies for thousands of years.

It is only in our recent history that the practice of meditation made its way to Western culture and has very quickly gained momentum in many places along with the introduction and practices of yoga and other Eastern healing practices.

The benefits of meditation are broad and far-reaching, not just in the awakening of the Kundalini energy, but for your overall well-being. Some, but certainly not all of the benefits, are listed below.

Reduction of stress and anxiety.

Helps in the improvement of your attention span and cognitive function.

Brings you into closer self-awareness.

Decreases heart rate and benefits blood circulation.

Dissolve aggressive or overpowering behavior tendencies.

Can help in the healing of addictive behaviors.

Can help with the aging process, maintain healthy, youthful vitality, memory, and mental health.

Has been known to produce feelings of kindness, compassion, and love for humankind.

Connects you to your breathing practice to align your chakras.

Brings you into closer alignment with your spiritual practice and divine energy.

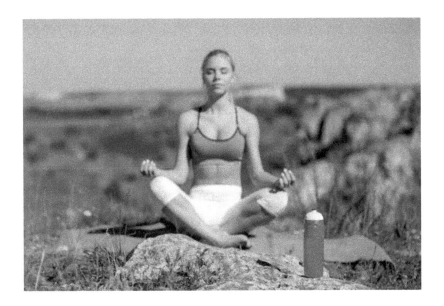

Helps with opening the third eye and creating a focus for psychic awareness and expansion. Again, these are just some of many of the benefits of meditation. It is an important component to the practice and experience of aligning and clearing your energy channels to allow for the balanced and synchronized flow of Kundalini.

If you have never meditated before, don't worry, you are not alone. It can feel foreign at first if you are not accustomed to doing it. Below is a simple approach to get you started.

Find a quiet place to sit comfortably. Do not worry if the space is not entirely silent. Part of the approach to meditation principles is to tune out the inner and outer noise and just be present in the here and now. Part of the 'here and now' includes noises and interruptions, so just breath through any distractions.

You can sit on a chair with your back straight and hands resting on your knees, or you can sit cross-legged on the floor. Try to find a position that you can sit in for a long stretch of time. Focus on breathing in and out. Try to focus only on your breath. You may start to feel distractions from the outside world (cars going down the street, your cat rubbing up against your leg, the telephone ringing) but all you have to do is return to your focus on your breath.

Keep your breathing long, deep and slow. Use your internal thought process to count as you breathe, in for five counts, out for five counts. Your mind may start to wander as well from your internal thoughts processing (Did I lock the car door? What should I eat for dinner? How long do I have to do this meditation thing?) If your mind starts to wander, just return to your breath, in for five counts, out for five counts.

Sit in this position for as little as five minutes, or as long as thirty or more. You can set a pleasant, or gentle, low volume timer to alert you to the end of your time frame, or just trust your intuition to stop you when you are ready.

At the end of your meditation time, simply open your eyes. Take a moment to mindfully take in the room, or space around you and re-engage with your daily life.

As you open yourself to regular meditation, you will be more open and available to empowering the Kundalini energy to rise within. It is not just one thing that helps activate this dormant energy, it is many. Creating your relationship to this energy by following the practices outlined in this book will help you find the spiritual enlightenment, self-awareness, and divine energy waiting to guide you into wholeness.

Chapter 6 Relaxing Your Inner Peace

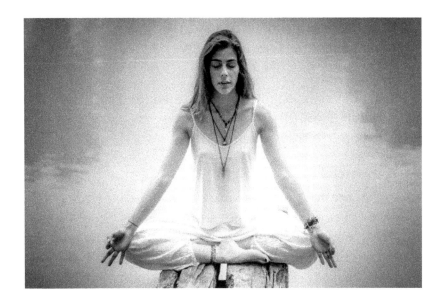

Practicing meditation regularly is important to your spiritual self and when trying to awaken Kundalini. What exactly is meditation? If you were to ask people what they thought meditation was, they would probably respond with a monk who spends hours sitting still with their eyes closed chanting and experiencing all sorts of things.

Technically, it is not either one of these. Meditation is how you train your mind. Meditation improves concentration and focus, stills your mind, and releases stress. There are several definitions you could give meditation.

Meditation can be used to awaken Kundalini, achieve enlightenment, and enhance psychic abilities. It can be found in many different spiritual practices and religions. It does not belong to any specific religion or group. Meditation can be performed by anyone.

It is hard to figure out what meditation is about without experiencing it in person. The best way to better understand it is to regularly practice it.

Before trying to meditate, there are some guidelines you need to keep in mind. This will help you meditate properly. Here are some to think about:

The spine needs to be straight

It does not matter what posture you are using, you need to constantly keep your spine straight. This is extremely important when meditating. The main reason to keep the spine straight is to make sure energy flows freely through all of the chakras. Keep in mind your chakras are located along your spine. When you can keep it completely straight, the energy will flow smoothly and freely. This is very important when trying to wake up Kundalini. Many people make the mistake of slouching while meditating. Before even attempting to meditate, you need to teach yourself how to have the correct posture.

When you are first starting out, you might find it hard not to slouch when sitting. Do not let this get you discouraged. By practicing a lot, your body will adjust and all of a sudden you will find that it is easy to do. So practice, practice, and practice some more.

Relax

When meditating, you need to be completely relaxed. Let your body completely relax and free your mind. Do not think that what you are doing is hard to do. This will put pressure on yourself that will keep you from reaching the higher state of consciousness. Relax and put all your focus on meditating. The more you pressure yourself, the more you will stay inside your physical body. Relax so you can become lighter. Once you are light, then you will be able to transcend into higher consciousness. The main thing to do is relax and let everything go.

Music

Music has a relaxing effect on our body. It helps us unwind. The choice of music is important; you should choose classical music pieces or musical soundtracks around the 432, 528 Hz frequency. Sounds of Tibetan bells can also be fine. The fundamental thing is that the sounds you choose as the background that you will then listen; have to please yourself to have a good result. Try different pieces of music until you find the right music for you.

Correct posture

When meditating, it is important to keep a correct posture. There are various ways you can meditate. You could meditate walking, standing, sitting, and even lying down. There are pros and cons in regards to each posture. If you meditate while laying down, you will be able to relax easier. One common problem when doing this position is you could fall asleep. This can be a problem for many beginners.

If you meditate while standing, you will find it a lot harder to fall asleep, and it will be hard to focus because you have to exert effort while holding this position.

This posture will get tiring. These reasons hold true when you meditate when walking. The most recommended posture when meditating is sitting.

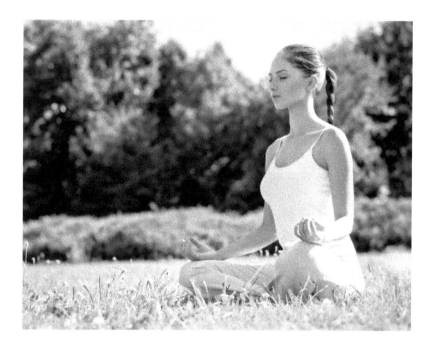

This allows you to be focused and awake. This is the main posture that most spiritual masters use. Buddha achieved enlightenment when meditating while sitting. You have the choice of meditating while sitting on the floor or a chair. When you are meditating on your bed or floor, you could put a pillow under your bottom to make you more comfortable.

You're safe

The main thing you need to know is that meditation is completely safe. There are some who think that meditating could place you in danger or even kill you. If you are not meditating when crossing the street or driving, then be assured you are going to be safe. According to gurus and people who are experienced in meditating, if your physical body is ever put in danger while meditating like if a fire were to break out, you will be brought back to your physical body immediately. While meditating, you don't have to worry about being safe. This will cause your attention to be divided. Put your entire focus on your meditation.

Most gurus will only teach the most important guidelines while meditating because if you have too much information, your mind might be tempted to wander. Now it is time to learn what meditation is truly about. Even if you do not see any changes, even to your state of mind, don't get discouraged. By practicing regularly, you will get better at meditating. Constant practice is the key.

Focus

While meditating, you are going to be asked to keep your focus on something. It might be an object or a sound. Do not let your mind wander. Remember what your focal point is and stick to it. If other thoughts come to mind, just ignore them and bring your focus back to that object.

The biggest challenge when learning to meditate is called the "monkey mind" which is the inability of your mind to be at rest. It is when your mind is completely full of thoughts. Just like a monkey will jump from branch to branch, so will your mind leap from one thought to another. When you are just learning how to meditate, you are going to face this challenge. How can you handle the monkey mind? There is just one way to control your monkey mind, and that is to constantly practice meditating. The more you practice, the more you will be able to make your mind stay still.

Basic Meditation

Your first meditation should be a simple breathing meditation. This is the most basic technique. Do not underestimate how powerful this meditation can be. Many monks, gurus, spiritual masters, and even Buddha practiced this meditation for many years. This meditation is powerful because of its simplicity. This is how to do the breathing meditation:

Sit in a relaxing position. Relax and start to take deep and slow breaths.

Focus on your breathing. Gently breathe in and breathe out as deeply as you can.

Slowly count to 3 in your mind while inhaling, hold your breath and count to 3 and then exhale slowly as you count to 3 in your mind.

Keep repeating this until this breathing rhythm becomes natural and you do not need to count. Continue this process for 3-5 minutes.

This technique can be done for however long you want. If you are a beginner, you may want to do this for only a couple of minutes. Some people who are experienced in meditating will do this meditation for hours. You only need to do this for whatever amount of time feels comfortable to you. It is not a good idea to rush your progress. Always try to do your best and stay committed. This simple meditation can empower and energize your chakras. Practicing this meditation allows you to reach a state of mind that will be completely new to you. When you are finished, you will be in a harmonious and peaceful state of mind.

Common Problems

There are several mistakes that could happen during meditation. You need to be aware of these problems so you can be sure not to commit them. Some of these problems cannot be avoided. Just do not get discouraged if some of these problems happen to you. Do your best and practice.

Wrong focus

While meditating, you can usually focus on either an object, sound or your breath. Some people will focus on focusing rather than focusing on a particular object while meditating. This may sound confusing but you have to understand this point. While meditating, do not tell yourself that you have to focus on specific objects. You cannot demand yourself to do it; you have to allow yourself to do it. Focusing calls for an action instead of a command. There is a huge difference between focusing on your breathing and demanding yourself to focus on breathing. You need to allow yourself time to reflect on this. Make sure you understand it completely.

Thinking

Meditation is not a time to start thinking. It is about doing. It is not about thinking about what is happening in this moment but just being present in the moment. While meditating, do not think, and just be present.

Another mistake is wondering if you are doing it right. If you have that thought going through your head, then you will meditate wrong. You may ask yourself this when the meditation is over but not while doing it. While meditating, you should never let yourself be divided.

Falling asleep

Most beginners make this mistake. Not to worry as this can be prevented. There are some points to remember. If falling asleep might become a problem, you should not meditate while lying down since this position could cause you to fall asleep.

You might also want to avoid meditating in your bed. Your bed might send a message to the brain that it is time to go to sleep. The best position is the sitting position. Try not to meditate when you are tired or right before going to bed. Most beginners who try to meditate before going to sleep will completely fall asleep. At this time, you are already exhausted and sleepy. You should try meditating during the morning when fully rested.

If you do not have any problems with going to sleep while meditating, then just ignore these measures. You can meditate whenever you feel like it. The best thing is to figure out what works for you.

Do not be hard on yourself. If you fall asleep, it usually means that you just need to rest. Just try again later.

Scratching

While meditating, you might feel like parts of your body are itching. Your automatic reaction is going to be to scratch it. The problem with that is your mind will take the focus away from the meditation and put it on your physical body. If you continue this, you will not be able to enter a deeper state of consciousness. Is there anything you can do about it? You will just have to ignore it. It is normal to get these sensations while meditating but you cannot let it distract you. This is hard to do at first, but you will eventually get used to it. After practicing enough, you will not be bothered by these sensations anymore. You will not even think about them. Just ignore them and go on. If you concentrate on them, they will distract you. Constant practice is what you need to do.

Being hard on yourself
Do not ever be too hard on yourself. Even if you think you cannot meditate the right way, be easy on yourself. When you get frustrated, it only makes your efforts counterproductive. Rather than beating yourself up, you need to relax and think about it gently and carefully. Find the mistakes you have been making and adjust things accordingly. You will meditate better if you are filled with positive energy and feel happy. Do not pressure yourself. Use energy to focus on your meditation and do the best you can. Remember that if you do your best, you might not be able to awaken Kundalini or become enlightened immediately. This will take effort, time, and practice. You need to appreciate that you are on the correct path and you are heading to mastery.

Not practicing enough
Learning how to meditate is like learning any new skill. It will take practice. Don't expect to do well if you only practice one day a week. If you are serious about your spiritual development, you need to make meditation a priority and do it daily.

If you are just beginning, you can do just five or ten minutes daily. As you get better, you can practice longer. Constant practice is imperative. You should make a schedule for meditating and stick with it. By doing this, you will make sure you have time to meditate. Without constant practice, it will be impossible to reach spiritual maturity.

Expectations

While meditating, you have to place your focus on a specific object. This means that you have to let go of any and all expectations. When you have expectations, it will only divide your energy. Having expectations will keep you from having 100 percent focus. Instead of creating expectations, you should relax and stick with your practice.

Chapter 7 Increasing Your Self-Worth

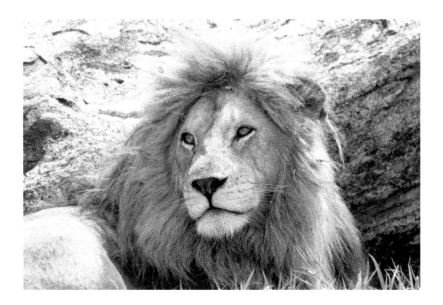

Now that we have a better understanding of Kundalini energy, chakras, and the third eye, let's look at the different ways through which this powerful life force or energy can be activated.

- Sit upright—It becomes easier to control your breath and breathe mindfully during the process of yoga and meditation if your spine is erect and your crown is pointed to the ceiling. Sit as tall as you can with your spine stature stacked. It will facilitate a better flow of energy and increase your chances of awakening Kundalini energy. Doing this effortlessly may entail first building up some core strength.

- Focus on your breath—Start by focusing intently on your breathing pattern. Concentrate on your breathing and focus on it as the inhaled air reaches the base of your spine, then direct it upwards slowly until it reaches your crown – then slowly exhale.

- Eliminate negativity—Attempt to get rid of negativity in all aspects of your life. It can be everything from removing accumulated physical clutter to negative people to destructive thoughts from your mind. A positive mind is a shelter for Kundalini awakening. Focus on positive attributes of your life, in every situation.

- Refine your food intake habits— "We are what we eat" is not a mere motivational statement to get us to eat right. If you are attempting to awaken an infinite and profound internal energy, complement your practice with nutritious, wholesome, plant-based, and holistic foods. It will influence your thoughts, mindset, physical health, and mood in several ways.

- Move—Unlocking dormant energy from the base of your spine involves showing your body nurturing and devotion. Be sure to put your body through a series of movements via an enjoyable daily exercise routine. It can be anything from a long walk in the woods to dancing to playing a fun sport. Anything that moves your body and gets you sweating can increase your chances of feeling positive and activating latent energy.

- Be a silent observer — We are the central characters in the play or movie of our own life, which means that we can never view events or circumstances happening to us in a detached manner. At times, learn to be a silent observer, even when everything seems to be working against you and the urge to react negatively is high. Rather than letting it affect you or dump a load of negative emotions over you, simply acknowledge it and allow it to pass. You'll feel much better emotionally and increase your ability to focus on activating the Kundalini energy.

- Look out for your tribe — On a subconscious level, we often mirror people we are surrounded by, which is why it is said that we are a reflection of the five people we spend the most time with. Opt to surround yourself with positive, compassionate, genuine, inspiring, supportive, and sensitive people. The quality of your life will be significantly impacted by the energy you receive from these people, which in turn will help you activate and tune in to your Kundalini more effectively.

- Chant — Few things can work up your energy vibrations like chanting. Chanting is known to be a highly positive and devotional practice that facilitates the right mood for helping us activate our dormant Kundalini. Find a saying, mantra, quote, or any positive words you feel comfortable and positive chanting and include them in your yoga or meditation practice.

- Activate your passions and interests — we are often going through life on autopilot mode, doing things without much thought because we have been subconsciously programmed to do so. Learn to make time for activities you enjoy or are passionate about. Set aside some time from your busy schedule to pursue activities you experience a close connection with, such as gardening, knitting, music, sports, art, and so on. Make activities that give you pleasure and fulfillment a priority.

Clearing the Blockages in Kundalini Awakening

Here are 7 ways that you can do to control your kundalini energy and enable it to rise smoothly: Treating Kundalini Syndrome Problems:

1. Be with Nature:

The fundamental objective as to establishing kundalini and lightening kundalini disorder manifestations needs to do with cutting down the vitality and bringing down the recurrence of its vibration.

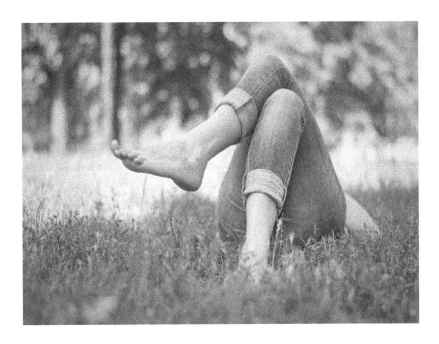

Some of what will be proposed will reflect what you would do when attempting to recuperate and adjust the Root Chakra, and in such manner, reconnecting with nature and earth is exceptionally useful.

Investing your time surrounding by nature particularly close trees and the earth, and you will find this experience extremely valuable in cutting down the awakening. Be as near to nature as you could be under the circumstances, so sitting up against trees or strolling bare feet on the grass is the thing that you ought to endeavor to do.

Similarly, planting or other gardening and landscaping activity which requires you to get your hands holding soil is a great way to get in touch with nature. Simple tasks such as weeding or even potting can get your hands dirty with soil so don't be afraid to explore. This will not only help your garden look great, but it will also clear any blockages and easy your kundalini rising.

2. Do Physical Work:

Again, the objective here is to get yourself connected with the earth and apart from being with nature, you can also start doing physical labor. If you feel your experience with kundalini is stunted, then you can do laborious tasks that get you sweaty. Physical work will help so try things like painting and carpentry, construction, building things or even cleaning up your house.

3. Do Physical Exercise:

Exercise as we know it has plenty of benefits. It makes your body more centered and oriented just like doing physical labor, but it also helps you fight anxiety that you may be feeling through your kundalini rising. The more you exercise - and this also includes doing yoga, you will feel more confident about your health and body and your body's alignment, and this also means you are less stressed and fearful about the changes happening to your body.

4. Eat Full Meals:

Part of clearing out any blockages is also having a good routine of eating. A regular and healthy diet is also key to a sound mind, heart, and body. Sometimes, it helps to eat bigger meals to deal with excessive kundalini energy. The goal here is to make your body more grounded to absorb any energy that rises, and it is also to keep you connected to earth and your life. Food is a strong connection to enable this.

5. Avoid Stimulants:

If you feel that your kundalini energy is out of control, you want to avoid stimulating it more. This is important because then this might cause a reaction that we are not ready for. For the time being, stay away from stimulants such as drugs, alcohol, tea, coffee, chocolates even.

6. Take a Break from Your Spiritual Practice:

Yes, it is true-taking a break from anything that you are overdoing is beneficial in the long run. The objective here is to not overstimulate your energy, so it is important to take a break from your spiritual practice until you feel better to handle the energy within you and the situation around you. This is a very personal decision to make so if you feel blockage then this would mean that your practice is out of balance and it needs to be re-evaluated. Too much of mantra of chakra meditation and not enough of physical yoga can throw you off balance and impinge on your spiritual activities. So best to stop, take a step back as this will greater benefit your practice and energy in the long run.

7. Rest and Relaxation:

Resting and relaxation give our body and our mind space and time it needs to absorb what we have done and learned and also heal. Overload of information or knowledge or exercise merely pulls us back instead of getting us forward.

Sometimes, it could also be that the kundalini energy is already working within you and a little bit of relaxation gives the energy a chance to do what it needs to do. Trust yourself and allow your body to take charge of cleansing and purifying itself.

At the end of the day, Kundalini is an extremely personal journey, and your experiences with the energy will be different from the next person. Listening to your own body is key because it allows you to hear what your heart needs as well. If the energy is too much, or there are blockages which you feel is preventing you from getting the full experience, then follow the guidelines above to help you get your flow back under control. It is a trial and error journey, going through the various ways to control energy within your body. Also, always look for help if you feel that these activities do not help.

Often time, speaking to someone-a guru or a yogi with more experience will help you find something that works for you.

Chapter 8 Building Strong Energy Within Your Mind And Body

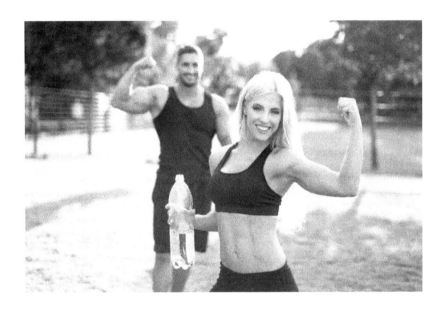

I n order to increase your chance of success, there are some practices you need to do every day.

Have the Correct Mindset

To progress on your spiritual journey, you have to think about spirituality. It is not the time for you to just see material things and how certain actions and things affect you. You need to think about how they affect you spiritually. If you have not been using your intuition, now is the time to begin paying attention to it and what it might be telling you. You have to be open to learn new things and change. If there is not any change, then there will not be any true improvements. Do not worry, since you should only change to be better. As your journey progresses, you will learn more about yourself. You have to be prepared to face your demons. If you get confused, just stick to what feels good for you.

Whatever you do, you need to give it everything you have. There are people that make up excuses not to give their best. They do this because they are afraid their best may not be good enough. Do not be like these people. You have not been defeated if you continue trying. If you are scared to do your best, then you have already been defeated. You have to always give your best and do not ever stop trying. You need to stay strong. Real strength is when your actions change with your entire soul and heart.

Take Breaks
Your spiritual path will be long and winding and you are going to face many challenges. This journey is not going to be fun if you are exhausted. You have to allow yourself time to take breaks. When you do take a break, do not think about spiritual matters. Let yourself totally relax and forget everything.

Constantly Practice
You should know by now that constant practice is the only way to have success. Be sure you meditate regularly. You do not have to do all the techniques in this book, but you need to choose one that you would like to master. Devote effort and time and practice it religiously. One problem many face is procrastinating and letting time go by without

learning anything new. Constant practice is the heart to spiritual progress. If you truly want to awaken Kundalini, you need to make constant practice your first priority.

Keep a Journal

This isn't a requirement but many people find writing in a journal is very helpful.

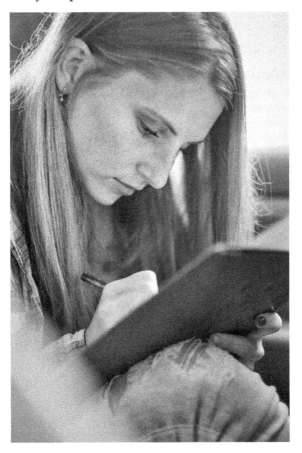

This allows you to look at yourself in different ways and lets you identify your weaknesses and strengths easier. Do not worry, you don't have to be a professional writer to be able to have a journal. You do have to keep it updated regularly.

You also need to be totally honest about everything that you write down in your journal.

The good thing about writing in a journal is you can write about anything that connects you to your spirituality. It needs to give the reasons why you have decided to take this path. It would be good to also include any mistakes and lessons you overcome along the way. This is your reflection about yourself on this spiritual path.

This is not just a tool for writing, but a way to learn when you reflect and read your writings. Make sure you take the time to read all your entries both past and present. Take time to reflect and learn from them. Try to get as much as possible out of it.

If you do not like writing, you could just create a word document on your computer. Many cell phones come with free writing apps on them, too. These make it easy and convenient to write in a journal daily. Make sure you do not delete any files or lose them. Most people prefer to use the classic notebook and pen.

Mistakes

You need to make sure you learn something from your mistakes. It does not matter how careful you are, you are going to make mistakes. Do not beat yourself up about it. Just learn from them. If you commit mistakes, take the time to think about them. Figure out how you can keep from making the same mistake in the future. What you need to understand is that each mistake is a lesson disguised to help you be a better person. The more you learn from your mistakes, you will improve and grow more.

Spirituality

It is totally normal when you go down a spiritual path to get lost every now and then. The most common cause is a person's greed. You might develop psychic abilities on this path even if you try to ignore them. Most people think that acquiring this power ends achievement. This is not the case. These powers are a part of a normal spiritual life. Do not get too attached. If you let these powers overtake you, you will get trapped and you won't discover how beautiful true spirituality is. Even waking up Kundalini is only a small part of your spiritual journey. It is important that you control yourself and stay focused on spiritual maturity and growth.

Sacrifice

There will be times on your spiritual path that you are going to make sacrifices. Let's say you go out with friends every Friday night, you might need to skip some of these and take time to meditate. This is not saying that your spiritual journey has to separate you from others. Instead, this is just saying that you need to remember your responsibilities if you want to make progress on your spiritual journey. It is like anything else in life that is worth having, you might have to make some sacrifices every now and then. Do not worry, the outcome of this journey is worth every bit of effort you put into it.

Chapter 9 Guided Meditation For Healing, Activating, And Balancing Chakras With Kundalini

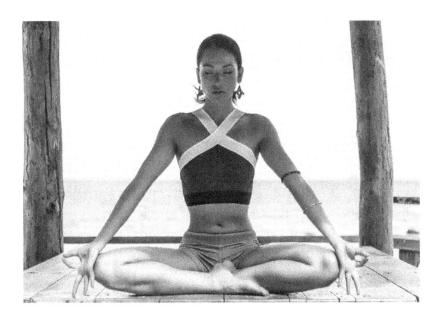

The meditation you are going to read in this section is a powerful awakening meditation that takes no more than about 15 minutes to complete. You can use this meditation to awaken your Kundalini energy and empower yourself to drop into your center for a balancing experience.

How To Use This Meditation

This awakening meditation should be used at least once per day. Using it first thing in the morning is a great way to awaken your Kundalini energy for the day. It also gives you the opportunity to balance your energies as you go on, allowing you to continue operating from a gentle and intentional life force flow.

This meditation requires a specific breathing pattern which will be outlined in the script below. As you use this breathing alongside the meditation in your daily practice, you will likely find that the new breathing rhythm becomes your natural breathing rhythm. As this happens, you can be sure that you are effectively infusing your daily life with Kundalini energy. As the energy is at work, this renewed breathing pattern will infuse naturally. Let it.

This meditation, as previously mentioned, should take approximately 15 minutes. It is easy to incorporate into your daily routine and can have a powerful effect on all that you do. It will help you destress, awaken, and approach your day in a powerful manner.

It is important that you realize that Kundalini awakening and meditation are both journeys. As such, you need to commit to using these practices on a daily basis.

This does not mean that you should feel shame or guilt if you miss a day. However, you want to do your best to refrain from missing any days. A truly awakened Kundalini energy will support you in remaining true to your practice day in and day out, which will allow you to continue to further awaken your energy. The more you commit, the more power you will gain from this practice.

"Begin by finding your center. You can do this by bringing your awareness to the tip of your nose, and then drop it straight down into the center of your body, where your solar plexus chakra resides. Once you have, begin using your breath as your center of focus. You want to block out the chatter in your mind by focusing entirely on rhythmic breathing. Right now is a great time to breathe deeply into your diaphragm, fill your lungs, and then fill your throat with air. As you exhale, empty your throat, then your lungs, and then your diaphragm. Continue doing this without pausing in between. Simply breathe. While you cannot ask your heart to beat at a different rate, breathing steadily in rhythmic breathing can help calm your heart center and bring your body into complete alignment and harmony.

As you continue breathing, begin breathing in a comfortable rate of four counts in… one, two, three, and four… and four counts out… one, two, three, and four. Keep this comfortable rhythm gently flowing through your lungs as you continue to keep your awareness on your center and your breath.

While you breathe, you may begin to recognize movement in your lower belly area. This signifies that it is time to awaken your energy. This movement is often noticed as a sensation or a fluttering of energy. You can recognize it by the way it feels, and by keeping your awareness on yourself and your inner world.

When you do, continue breathing with your count of four. Let the energy begin to arise, coming up your spine. This rising energy comes from your sacral chakra and continues to flow up your spine, purifying it with life force energy. Rather than visualizing it, simply become aware of the process as it happens.

Stay focused on the energy rising, and set the intention to draw it all the way up your spine. Continue letting it rise until it reaches the crown of your head.

Breathe here for a few moments. In, two, three, four... out, two, three, four...

And as the process completes itself, take a few moments to relax and settle into the sensations that come with it. Then, when you are ready, draw your awareness back to the room and awaken yourself to the life around you. Take a few moments to feel how the sensation continues to reside within you, despite the fact that you are now awakened to the energy of the room. Carry this energy with you throughout your day, allowing it to be infused with all that you do. Let it inspire you, guide you, and continue to awaken you as you move throughout your daily routines."

Balancing and Clearing Your Energetic Channels and Centers

There are times that although we practice kundalini and it's supposed to make us more energetic, on the other hand, we feel the exact opposite. We feel like an emotional drain, feeling groggy and less vital. If this is happening to you right now, it could that you have your chakra clogged.

Chakra is not some new age terms-it is an ancient system of understanding our body's energy the channel of which kundalini energy flows. As we know, these chakras in our body are located in the energetic spine's central channel which yogic texts call sushumna. This is a major channel that energy flows (Nadi) through is located at the base of our spine running all the way to the top of our head or the crown. Where are these chakras located in our body and how do we know if they are clogged?

The image above shows where exactly our chakras are located, and in previous chapters, we described what each of these meant and how it relates to our body and what it controls or oversees.

How to Get Your Energy Flowing

Whenever you feel that your energy is stuck in a specific chakra, these tips below will help get your energy flowing again:

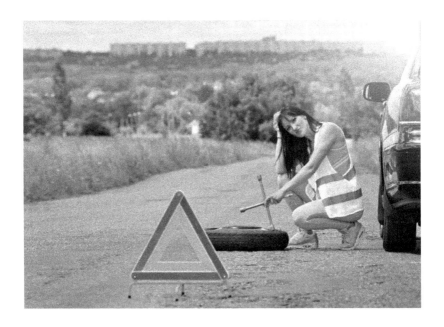

1st Chakra (Root)

Element: This chakra is connected to the earth. Walking barefoot on the ground, allowing sand to get between your toes is beneficial. Time spent in nature will revive this chakra.

Nutrition: Eat foods that are red such as beets, tomatoes, berries, and apples.

Objects: Wear or use red jewelry, shoes and red clothing

Sound: lam

2nd Chakra (Sacral)

Element: This chakra is associated with water, so spending time near bodies of water is ideal. Swimming in oceans and lakes is also beneficial.

Nutrition: Connect back by eating foods rich in carotenes like oranges and carrots melons, or mangoes.

Objects: Wear or use or be around objects that have orange tones whether a scarf, earrings or even a ring.

Sound: vam

3rd Chakra (Solar Plexus)

Element: The element of fire is associated with the solar plexus chakra. Soaking up the son, being outdoors in sunlight or even sitting around a campfire or bonfire is beneficial.

Nutrition: Consuming food that is rich in the color yellow such as pineapples, bananas, turmeric, ginger, and corn will help

Objects: Wearing yellow clothing, jewelry, and accessories will unblock this chakra.

Sound: ram

4th Chakra (Heart)

Elements: The heart chakra relates to air, so deep breathing meditations and exercise helps clear this chakra. Alternatively, flying a kite, driving with the windows down and taking a boat ride would also help.

Nutrition: Eat loads of leafy green foods such as kale, spinach and of course broccoli and avocado.

Objects: Green is your ultimate friend here so accent your life with green objects.

Sound: yum

5th Chakra (Throat)

Element: This chakra, the throat chakra relates to ether, so simple things like sitting in an open field under a clear blue sky is a great way of opening up this chakra. This also helps open up the third chakra too.

Nutrition: your meal times should consist of blue colored foods such as blueberries and currants, kelp and grapes and eggplant.

Objects: Accessorize with blue accents from ties to belts, earrings to pendants.

Sound: ham

6th Chakra (Third Eye)

Element: The third eye chakra is connected to the light. To open and balance this chakra, sit under sunlight or where there is natural light pouring in. As much as possible, allow natural light to touch you on a daily basis.

Nutrition: anything indigo here is good from grapes, blackberries, purple cabbage, purple yam, and figs.

Objects: Indigo or purple clothing and jewelry is your best friend so color your life with accents of purple from vases to curtain, earrings to rings, necklaces and ties.

Sound: sham

7th Chakra (Crown)

Element: The crown chakra is associated with wholesomeness which is all the elements. You need to connect with all elements as opposed to just one single element here. To do this, you need to spend time in chanting, praying and meditation directed to unblocking the crown chakra.

Nutrition: With the crown chakra, it is not about the physical body anymore rather, the spiritual being. Self-reflection is best to practice at this point as this chakra is not nourished by food rather with curiosity and self-help.

Wear and Decorate: Wearing violet clothing or jewelry and decorating with accents of this color helps connect this chakra.

Sound: OHM

Chapter 10 Powerful Easy Techniques For Awakening The Body's Complex Kundalini Energy

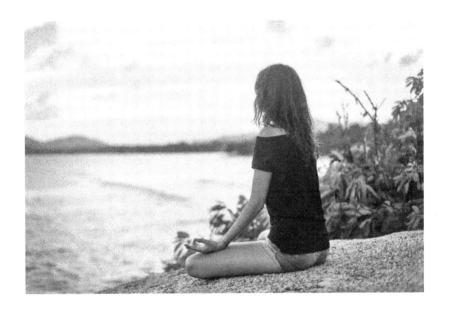

Here is the first technique for awakening your dormant kundalini energy to enjoy its innumerable benefits. This is not guided meditation in its strictest sense, but more of a focused technique for activating the body's Kundalini energy.

Relax your body completely and breathe softly to prepare through breathing. Ensure you are wearing comfortable clothes and are seated in a comfortable position in a calm and distraction-free space. Slowly close your eyes now.

Use soft abdominal breathing patterns. Experience the flow of fresh oxygen into your throat, lungs, heart, and abdomen. This is the simplest way to identify the hidden energy pathway. When we inhale, the expanding lungs push into the abdomen (diaphragm) and subsequently into the pelvic organs.

Allow your lungs to achieve a state of equilibrium with your diaphragm, moving gently together.

Identify your kidneys. They are located slightly behind the membrane in the space between the two the airbags of your lungs and diaphragm. Now, connect to your kidneys with each inhalation, and subsequently release both these airbags together as you exhale. This will end up massaging your kidneys. Do not open your eyes.

Note your adrenal glands next to the kidneys. Begin chanting "Num Mum Yum Pa'Hum." Let the bags come into contact with each other as you inhale. When you exhale while chanting, closely tune in to the vibration experienced in the right adrenal, the right kidney, the left adrenal, and the left kidney. Come into your body and experience a sense of oneness with the present moment.

Rub throughout your lower back and ribs with the back of both your palms if you are still experiencing pain in them or they feel stuck. Avoid sitting in a rigid position and eliminate all discomfort.

Raise both your arms over your head, stretch your thumbs while rotating your arms back out. Consciously experience your lungs responding to signals received through the thumbs. Raise your index finger in the direction of the sky while allowing the large intestine to hang from your ribcage.

Raise your collarbones and stretch from your collarbones to your dangling kidneys, followed by pressing and rotating the ball of each of your feet. Draw your awareness to the two airbags again. Experience the sensation in these two airbags and in-between the kidney and adrenal.

Begin to release the diaphragm but do not exhale everything at once. Simply stick your chin out slightly and create a gentle position of the throat that helps it lead you into slow exhalation.

Now inhale, touch the two bags of lungs and diaphragm, while resting the palate, chin, sinuses, and tongue above the spinal stack, along with your third bag - the bag of the spinal cord and brain.

Slowly exhale while feeling your lungs filled and floating upwards. Visualize developing wings with every exhalation, and imagine the wing rising above the lungs to keep you going.

Inhale and make contact with the pleural chest bag to the bag of abdomen and pelvis. Exhale slowly and allow the third (spinal or dural) bag to rise above the top of your nose.

Start breathing again and let your dural bag expand just under the inner realms of the top of the dome inside your head. Allow the spinal cord bag to rise from the spine and backbones. Start your hunt for the hidden pathway into the central energy channel.

Think of yourself as a musical instrument as you continue chanting. You are an instrument that spreads joy. You are receiving love, compassion, and kindness from every direction.

Chant "Shum Shum Shum Shum." You will experience the vibration of this chant throughout the sacrum bone. Tune in to the craniosacral wave beginning to rise from the spine.

Experience the third bag filled with fluid surging up and later settling down again. Allow your brain to slowly sink into the water there. Let it float gradually.

Visualize a balloon that is as big in size as the abdomen and pelvis airbag. Release air from the balloon slowly, holding the mouth of the balloon and gradually stretching it. This will let you point the tiny jet of air wherever you desire.

Lift your pelvic area slightly and squeeze your anal sphincters enough to experience or imagine a ring. These are muscles that manage the nozzle and stream of air as you breathe out. Allow the two airbags to come into contact with each other through soft inhalation. Feel the kidneys juxtaposed between the two bags and allow the chin to rest over the air.

Now, draw the third brain bag forward slightly while lifting your spinal cord gradually. Raise your pelvic floor, engage your spinal base sphincter rings and begin to exhale gradually.

Now, blow the abdominal balloon jet backward from the frontal hollow of your upper sacrum along the lower spine.

Look for the hidden passage to the central energy channel. Look for it all the way to the insides of your belly button and lower back. Place both your palms on your belly and feel a tingle.

Push in and perform a complete exhalation cloud within the central energy channel.

If you think you've activated a hidden latch, or if there's any uncertainty, move your head upwards while keeping your eyes firmly shut.

Push through the wall if you come against one. If you spot a road, drive through it. Keep looking up. Inhale and then rest your bags.

Engage your pelvic muscles. This time, exhale from the left side in the direction of your midline located just under the navel. Repeat it a few times. Chant "Bum Ba'Hum Mum Yum Rum Lum." These are sounds connected to six petals of the Svadhisthana lotus chakra. Move from the right lower abdomen to your appendix to your right kidney and then to the left kidney, left colon, and finally, the left ovary.

Chant "Lum Lum Lum Lum," which asks for the grace of the universal forces or almighty. Inhale and from the left end, exhale towards the central focal line. Inhale while allowing the three bags to rest.

Bring down your awareness through the spine. Visualize the sound of "H" while exhaling, allow your lower abdominal region to move quickly.

Visualize doing something like flipping a bread or pancake.

Exhale forward up and allow it to loop around with the small jet blowing before the abdomen wall. It goes through the wall and the way to the frontal area of the spinal column. If you feel itchy, exhale all over again, very slowly, moving towards your final goal of equilibrium.

Exercise 1 – Crow Pose

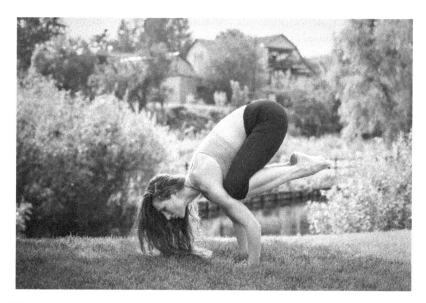

Time: 5 minutes

For this exercise, lay down a yoga mat or find a carpeted area. To begin, squat down with your feet flat on the ground. Extend your arms straight ahead, clasping hands together while pointing with both index fingers. Stare straight down the line of your arms and focus directly ahead of you. Begin Breath of fire; rapid breathing through the nose, allowing your stomach to extend while inhaling and withdraw while exhaling sharply. Continue this fast-paced breathing while holding the crow position as long as you can. Once finished, break the crow pose by placing your hands on the ground behind you and slowly moving back on to your knees with your feet behind you raised by your toes. Extend your arms in the crow pose once more while remaining on your knees and the edge of your toes. Clasp your hands in front of you and point with your index fingers while staring straight ahead into infinity. Begin Breath of fire once more, sharply inhaling and exhaling through your nose. If you need a small break, you may breathe deep slow instead of the fast-paced breath of fire practice. Continue for one minute.

Repeat the exercise for up to ten minutes, but do not push yourself. Always listen to your body and work at your own pace.

Exercise 2 – Mandukasana

This exercise focuses on stretching the inner thighs and groin area; so do not push yourself beyond your bodily limits. This action stimulates both our first Muladhara chakra and then our second chakra, Svadhishthana. Only do what is comfortable for you. If you have sensitive knees, it would be best to use pillows or even a folded blanket underneath the knees to relieve pressure.

To begin, in a seated position with your feet below your knees, exhale deeply while rolling your spine forward and over your legs. Press your big toes together and then slowly begin to walk your knees apart only as far as they will comfortably allow. While keeping your big toes together, slowly push the inside edges of your feet to the edges of your yoga mat. If your toes separate, the frog pose will be broken. Keep them together as much as you possibly can and make sure the angle of both your knees and hips does not exceed 90 degrees.

Sink your pelvis slowly to the floor while stretching your neck forward and keeping your gaze pointed downwards. Exhale and allow your chest to lower to the ground, opening the joints in your hips. Keep your weight pressed into your elbows while relaxing your stomach and heart. Allow your shoulder blades to draw back while making sure to push your hips downwards and back.

Exercise 3 – Leg and Core Poses

Exercise: Alternate Leg Lifts, Cat-Cow Pose, Cobra Pose, Boat Pose

Time: 40 minutes

Gently lay back so that your back is flat on the ground. Place your arms parallel to your body, folding your hands behind your back if extra support is needed. Take a deep inhale while slowly lifting your right leg straight above you at a ninety-degree angle. Keep your feet flexed to ensure a more thorough stretch through your muscles. Hold your leg in this position for ten seconds while being sure not to rotate or strain your opposite side. Upon exhaling, lower your leg back to the ground and pause for a moment to relax your body. Next, lift your left leg up at a ninety-degree angle, flex your toes forward, and hold for another ten seconds. Repeat this alternate leg lift exercise for fifteen more reps of each side.

Once finished, carefully push yourself up into a sitting position with your legs extended straight in front of you. Place your hands back so that they are just behind your hips. Lift your weight to the top of your sternum and lean your back slightly backward, making sure not to curve the spine in the process. Exhale slowly and bend your knees, lifting your feet off the floor so that your thighs are at fifty-degree angles. If possible, slowly straighten your knees while stretching so that your toes raise just above your eye level. If this is too difficult, keep your knees bent so that your shins are parallel with the floor.

Stretch your arms along the side of your legs so that they are parallel to each other and the floor. Spread your shoulder blades across your back and extend your fingers as far forward as you can. If this stretch proves to be too much as well, keep your hands either at your sides next to your hips, or hold on to the backs of your thighs.

Hold your abdomen firm but do not overstrain your muscles. Try your best to keep your stomach as flat as you can while holding this position. Press the heads of your thighbones towards the floor to help anchor your sternum in place. Take deep and steady breaths in this completed Boat Pose. Stay in this pose for ten to twenty seconds on your first try before relaxing and trying again for a slightly longer amount of time. To release correctly, lower your legs upon exhalation and sit back upright once you inhale again.

Shift your position so that you are instead sitting with your legs behind you and resting on top of your heels. Slowly lean forward on to all fours with your hands aligned with your shoulders and your knees aligned with your hips. Begin the Cat-Cow Pose by beginning with the cow; slowly inhale while lowering your abdomen and rolling your neck back and tailbone upwards. Hold this position for a moment before exhaling and reversing the position by pulling your stomach back and arching your back like a cat with head and tailbone tilting downward. Keep your arms and legs straight through both poses and continue for fifteen more reps, making sure to take deep slow breaths.

Next, carefully lower yourself to the ground so that you are lying flat on your stomach with legs straight behind you and arms parallel to our sides. Take a moment to relax your muscles and recover your breathing if needed.

When ready, slowly bring your hands forward so that your palms are flat on the floor underneath your shoulders and hug your elbows into your body. Press the tops of your feet, thighs, and lower abdomen into the floor while slowly pushing yourself upwards with your arms. Gently curl your spine backward to lift your chest off the floor while keeping your chin parallel to the ground. Make sure to lift through the top of your sternum, being careful not to strain yourself. Flatten your shoulder blades along your back while puffing your side ribs forward. Avoid as best you can from pushing your frontal ribs forward, as this will only harden our lower backs, causing us strain. Make sure to feel the stretch evenly through your entire spine. Hold this pose before slowly lowering yourself back to the ground in a resting position. Repeat the stretch several more times before carefully pushing yourself back into a comfortable sitting position.

Exercise 4 – Core Balancing
Time: 30 minutes

Sit comfortably on top of your yoga mat or a carpeted surface. Create the Shuni Mudra with each hand by touching the tip of your ring finger to your thumb while keeping your other three fingers extended and relaxed. Begin with whistle breaths by gently creating a small 'o' with your mouth and then inhale creating a high pitched sound before exhaling through your nose. Repeat this breathing style fifteen times before alternating to inhale through your nose and creating a high-pitched whistle while exhaling through your mouth. Continue this for another fifteen full reps.

Next, shift to sit with your legs crossed. Break the Shuni Mudra and switch to the mudra of the Ego Eradicator by curling your fingers so that the tips touch their base joints and extend your thumbs upwards, stretching them as far back from your fingers as you can. Keep your back and neck straight while slowly extending your arms up along your sides that they raise up alongside your head at a forty-five-degree angle.

Repeat breath of fire for another two minutes. Gently break the pose of the Ego Eradicator by slowly lowering your arms and relaxing both of your hands. Inhale slowly, pause, and exhale.

Next, comfortably shift your sitting position so that both of your feet are pressed flat against each other in front of you. Make sure that you join your toes, heels, and balls of your feet together. Place both of your palms on the tops of your feet and continue to push your feet more completely together while being careful not to pull them upwards towards yourself. Keep your spine straight and your chin level with the floor. Take a deep, slow inhale through your nose and gently lift both of your knees up towards your shoulders. Upon exhaling, slowly lower your knees back down and curl your neck and shoulders forward. Inhale once more, curling your spine upright once more while gently lifting your knees back up towards your shoulders. Make sure to keep your mind on your hands as well so that they are not grasping your feet too tightly. Once you reach back to your seated height with your back straight, gently begin to flutter both of your knees up towards your shoulders and then back towards the ground. While continuing this motion, make sure that you are not pulling up on your toes but instead still holding your feet gently together. Inhale deeply and pause before completely exhaling while continuing the fluttering motion with your legs. This completes the Butterfly Pose.

Next, carefully shift so that you may lie flat on your back with arms at your side and palms touching the floor. Keep your feet flat on the floor so that your knees are bent upward, making sure to align your feet with your hips. Take a deep inhale while slowly lifting your hips so that your thighs align with the rest of your torso. Hold this position for three seconds before exhaling and gently lowering your hips back to the ground. This action completes one rep of Pelvic Lifts. Continues this exercise for up to thirty more reps or, if you are experiencing too much strain, half the exercise to fifteen reps instead. Make sure that you keep your breathing steady, inhaling with each rise of the hips, and exhaling as you lower back down. Make sure to keep your abdomen and thighs firm so that your back does not arch or sink while you are holding your lifted position.

Once finished, gently lift your legs up towards your body so that they are folded on top of your abdomen. Place your palms on the front of your shins and gently hold, inhaling deeply and pausing before exhaling completely. Release your legs and lift them slightly so that your knees are directly above your hips while spreading your arms in a cross position with palms pressing into the floor. Take a gentle inhale and exhale while slowly rotating your hips to the right so that your bent legs are resting with the right against the ground and the left directly on top of it. Pause for a moment and feel the stretch down your spine while keeping your back as straight and flat against the ground as possible. Inhale once more and carefully bring your legs back upright, returning to your previous position of knees bent above the hips. Exhale and instead rotate your hips to the alternate side so that your left leg presses against the ground with the right resting on top.

Repeat this motion for thirty more complete reps, rotating the hips and legs from left to right. Focus on your breathing and make sure to go at your own pace so that you do not strain yourself.

Chapter 11 Philosophy of The Third Eye And How Awakening It Can Transform Your Entire Life

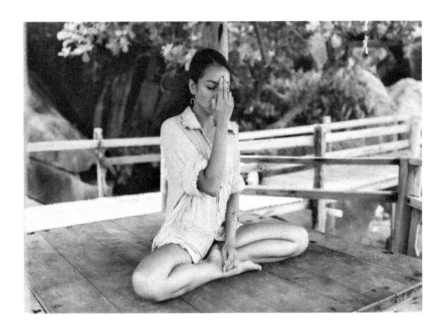

What is the Third Eye?

The pineal organ is a pea-sized organ molded like a pine cone, situated in the vertebrate cerebrum close to the nerve center and pituitary organ. Otherwise called the third eye, it is a worshipped instrument of soothsayers and spiritualists and viewed as the organ of

ENERGY HEALING

preeminent all inclusive association. Its centrality shows up in each old culture all through the world. For instance, in Ayurvedic reasoning, the third eye is spoken to by the Ajna chakra and in Ancient Egypt, the image of the Eye of Horus reflects the situation of the pineal organ in the profile of the human head. The third eye is associated with clearness, focus, creative mind and instinct.

Ever considered how to open your third eye, home to your "intuition?" Your instinct and higher astuteness wake up when this vitality focus is completely open and adjusted. Tragically, for a large portion of us, building up our third eye chakra and its capacities is trying, best case scenario, and may even now and again appear to be distant. Here are a couple of straightforward advances and suggestions to help.

Proven methodologies for arousing the third eye

To start with, we will portray the most significant rules that will assist you with building up your third eye.

Develop quietness

Cultivate the quiet of the brain, regardless of whether it's through reflection, simply sitting smoothly in nature, or being caught up in your preferred workmanship or game practice.

Why? Since third eye discernment hoists your faculties to increasingly unobtrusive levels. Some call it "the space in the middle of", mystic capacities, the domain of the undetectable.

To have the option to tune in to the messages and data that gets through your third eye, you ought to be prepared to see the murmur of its insight. On the off chance that your

249

psyche is occupied or boisterous, you may miss its primary message.

Sharpen your instinct

There are numerous approaches to develop your instinct. The third eye is the focal point of understanding, vision, and higher insight. So shouldn't something be said about getting to know your fantasies and their implications, maybe checking out at clear dreaming, becoming acquainted with how to peruse a horoscope or tarot cards? Find better approaches to intuit into your day by day life exercises.

Why? Since the third eye is the primary seat of more elevated levels of recognition and instinct. One approach to see it very well may be "phony it until you make it." at the end of the day, be interested, find out about these instinctive methods.

In time, these generally recondite practices will show up increasingly natural, and you will acquire trust in your very own capacities.

You don't have to pay attention to this – really, the inverse is prescribed. Have a ton of fun, investigate, and above all, keep your brain and chakras open to plausibility and marvel.

Make each cell in your body stir and cheer!

A large portion of us have fiery squares and awkward nature just as vitality attacking propensities that keep us from getting to our full imperativeness, which drives us to feel depleted, dissipated, dull… even sick.

Sustain your inventiveness

Let your inventiveness stream uninhibitedly by concentrating on explicit exercises or allowing your creative mind to imagination. For example, start learning another craftsmanship or art; don't attempt to be great, simply let your motivation go through your hands and be fit to be amazed by the outcomes.

Why? Innovativeness is an effective method to relax your sane personality – you know, the psychological babble that remarks each progression you make to see whether it's set in stone, that will in general control each activity with a particular plan and planned result.

At the point when you quiet the piece of your mind that needs to be accountable for how reality ought to be and use your innovativeness to open up conceivable outcomes, your third eye limit has more space to unfurl and bloom.

Ground yourself to all the more likely take off
For the greater part of us, it probably won't be evident that so as to open our third eye capacities, we have to initially land both our feet on the ground. Likewise note the significance of opening up continuously, building solid establishments first that will enable you to have legitimate insight and decipher your extrasensory recognitions with however much clearness as could be expected.

Why? Since we have to have enough vitality going through our entire body and fiery framework to help a sound opening of inconspicuous channels of recognition. At the point when the third eye gets enacted, the data that comes through might show up rather abnormal, new, or just upsetting to the basic personality.

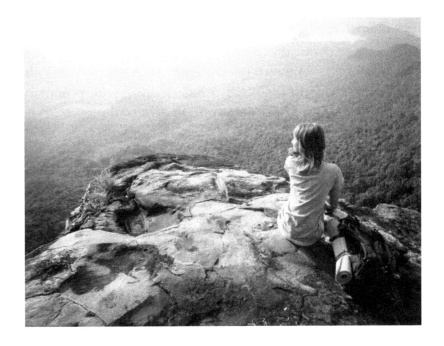

Being grounded and having enough vitality enables us to venture into unobtrusive elements of discernment. It can assist us with opening up unhindered and stay away from the basic negative indications of third educational, for example, feeling muddled or befuddled.

Importance of the Third Eye

Building up the third eye is the entryway to everything mystic — clairvoyance, special insight, clear dreaming and astral projection. The dream of division among self and soul disintegrates when the third eye association is developed. Magical methods for being are associated with the third eye, for example, how to be wakeful inside the fantasy, to stroll among substances and outperform the restrictions of humankind.

How Does Calcification Occur?

The calcification of the pineal organ is normal if the third eye isn't being utilized or because of diets wealthy in fluoride and calcium. Calcification is the development of calcium phosphate precious stones in different pieces of the body. This procedure happens on account of poisons in ordinary items, similar to fluoride, hormones and added substances, sugars and fake sugars. Radiation from mobile phone use and electric and attractive fields may affect the pineal organ also. Some connivance scholars accept broad crusades upholding the utilization of fluoride and calcium are spurred by government control programs.

Task: Celebrate the Third Eye

Most creatures have pineal organs, frequently bigger than human pineal organs, that drive instinctual information. While your pineal organ might be disregarded and decalcified, commend that you for sure have a pineal organ. Start your enactment practice essentially by sending appreciation to your third eye for your intrinsic instinctive capacities and your association with nature through the circadian rhythms that the pineal organ administers.

Go through 10 minutes every day deliberately initiating your third eye through contemplation, reciting, petition, move or yoga.

Third eye montage

Six Ways to Awaken Third Eye

Through decalcification and enactment, recover your way to happy euphoria and association with source:

Keep away from Fluoride

Give close consideration to the water in your life: faucet water is a wellspring of fluoride, which adds to pineal organ calcification. Fluoridated toothpaste is another conspicuous wellspring of fluoride in current weight control plans, as are inorganic produce and counterfeit beverages made with polluted water. Consider adding water channels to your sink and shower fixtures.

Supplement Your Diet

The rundown of enhancements that help and detoxify the third eye is long and incorporates crude cacao, goji berries, garlic, lemons, watermelon, bananas, nectar, coconut oil, hemp seeds, cilantro, ocean growth, nectar, chlorella, spirulina, blue green growth, crude apple juice vinegar, zeolite, ginseng, borax, Vitamin D3, bentonite mud and chlorophyll are generally fixings that helper filtration of the pineal organ.

Use Essentials Oils

Numerous fundamental oils invigorate the pineal organ and encourage conditions of otherworldly mindfulness, including lavender, sandalwood, frankincense, parsley and pine. Fundamental oils might be breathed in legitimately, added to body oil, consumed in a diffuser and added to bathwater.

Sungaze

The sun is an extraordinary wellspring of intensity. Look tenderly at the sun during the initial couple of moments of dawn and most recent couple of minutes of dusk to support your pineal organ.

Contemplate and Chant

Reflection initiates the pineal organ through goal: consider imagining the decalcification of the pineal organ, as its sacrosanct nature is lit up and straightforwardly associated with source. Reciting causes the tetrahedron bone in the nose to reverberate, which causes incitement of the pineal organ. Considering reciting "Om," otherwise called the sound of the universe, multiple times every day.

Allow Your Intuition To sparkle

When you start working with your third eye, you will start to get direction messages and dreams. Endeavor to have the mental fortitude to finish on what your instinct offers and your third eye quality will just develop.

Third Eye Awakening: How to Recognize If Your Sixth Chakra Is Open

At the point when the third eye arousing occurs, there are some striking impacts on your reasoning and feeling.

The third eye (otherwise called the inner consciousness arranged between your eyebrows) is the 6th chakra with amazing capacities. Generally, this region or chakra becomes dynamic when the individual has arrived at a specific degree of mindfulness and awareness.

When that the individual has empathy, love, trustworthiness and duty, at that point the third eye opens and uncovers better approaches for self-advancement.

In the event that you need to know whether your third eye is conscious, here you have 4 signs that will assist you with remembering it:

1. Instinct

On the off chance that your 6th chakra is opened, the principal ability you will acquire is instinct. You will have the option to determine what, how or when something will occur before it really does. It is an unpretentious inclination that will manage you and which will grow more and better with time.

2. Diverse reasoning

You search for personal growth and you start embracing an alternate reasoning. You fire abandoning old propensities, old demeanor and you need a psychological and otherworldly advancement. You start pondering your life or life itself, you start addressing what you know or what you hear/see.

You start breaking down and scanning for better approaches for advancement – either society improvement or self-awareness. You never again acknowledge a variant of an answer, yet you look for reality and need to know more.

3. A receptive outlook

Your third eye arousing enables you to comprehend complex circumstances or ideas which before might have been unreasonably muddled for you. You start seeing a circumstance from numerous edges and you can comprehend its various perspectives. You are likewise ready to convey your emotions and considerations easily.

4. Seeing outside of the crate

Your reasoning is never again molded by what individuals or broad communications let you know. You see through words and you can get the genuine significance/purpose for activities. You are in contact with your faculties, with life, with nature and you can comprehend the concealed messages you get from them (for example synchronicity).

Chapter 12 Opening Your Heart Chakra Through Anahata Stimulation

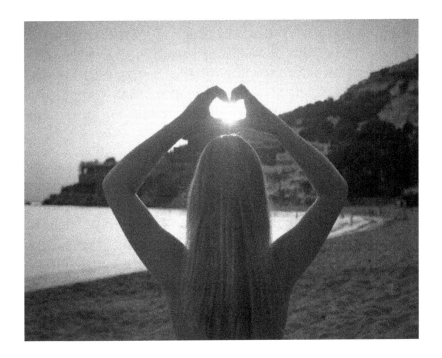

Heart Chakra: Anahata

The heart chakra brings the element of air. Air is all around us. You breathe it in and let some out. It changes the weather and cleanses out old, stagnant energy with one gust. To work with this energy and help clear and balance the heart chakra, find ways to get closer to this element. When you drive your car, turn off the air conditioner and drive with the wind in your hair. When you sleep at night, crack some windows and allow the fresh morning air to gently blow in while you wake up for a new day.

If you are comfortable and are able to go even further, take a boat ride so you can feel some fresh air on your face as you coast around the water, or try paragliding to really put some wind in your sails. At the very least, adopt a daily practice, morning and night, of healthful breathing exercises. They can be a part of your morning meditations, or evening yoga practice. You can also just breathe. Take some time throughout the day to stop whatever you are doing, and mindfully focus on your breath.

Eat green! There are tons of foods that are green and not only is it good to focus on this food color while you are healing your heart; it's also just great to eat a lot of vegetables, which so many green foods are. Some ideas for green foods to add to your heart chakra healing are broccoli, avocado, kiwi, kale, leafy greens, Brussels sprouts, spinach, herbs like rosemary, basil and thyme, green apples, bok choy, and so much more. Do your best to steer clear of processed foods, artificial colors, and sweeteners, alcohol and lot of caffeine.

Make your heart altar in the color green. Use green candles and anything you like that has this color. You can collect things from nature that are green or use green stones and crystals. Some of these for the heart chakra is green calcite, rose quartz, malachite, jade, rhodonite, and green aventurine. You can also wear these on your person as their energy will help remove blockages and create balance. Wear them with your green outfits or accent colors.

Bringing more of the color green into your life can also involve adding some new, luscious potted plants into your house. When you build your altar, put it with all of your houseplants so you have all the greenery in one place while you devote your attention to your heart chakra.

Sit among all the green and place your hand over your heart. Breath in and out several times, deeply. Breath in loving thoughts and energy, breathe out negativity held in the heart.

Say aloud or in the mind-heart healing affirmations such as:

I love myself unconditionally.

I forgive myself fully.

I am open to giving and receiving love.

I deserve to love and be loved.

I am worthy of healthy and loving relationships.

You can say this every day, or multiple times a day to really help your energy clear here. So many of us have large blocks in our heart chakra. An open heart is so important to fully awaken your Kundalini power.

For even more opening, intone the heart chakra sound, "yum." Put your hands over your heart as you intone this sound and feel the vibration of "yum" in your chest.

Mantras, Meditation, and Maintaining Your Practice

By this point in your understanding of Kundalini awakening, you know a significant amount about the chakras and energies within that require cleansing and balancing in order for your divine life-force to awaken and rise.

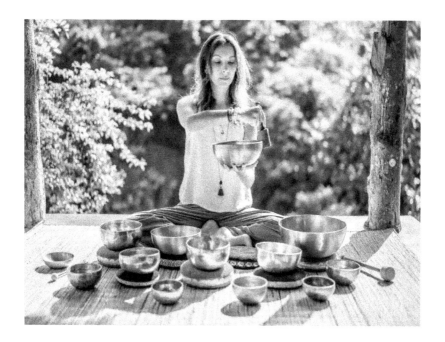

Mantras and meditations have similar value in the awakening process. So, what are mantras? That word, intoned either in the mind or aloud, is a mantra.

There are many mantras utilized across all the different yoga practices and Eastern healing philosophies, just as there are equally as many different meditations.

Meditations establish powerful changes in the way you think, your neural chemistry, and your emotional balances, whereas mantras bolster and reinforce those alterations made through meditating.

Mantras are small words, or phrases that encompass very big thoughts and ideas. The brain is open to the simple, rhythmic effect of these intonations and can have a powerful impact on your energy connection and your connection to divinity.

There are three ways that you can chant a mantra:

Normal to loud voice - This is the sound volume of humans, things and animals of the earthly, worldly plane.

Strong Whisper - This sound belongs to love and lovers, to the sense of belonging.

Silent - Mental language is the language of infinity.

There are several key mantras for Kundalini awakening, but to get you started, below are some to utilize in your emerging healing practices.

Sat Nam - This mantra means 'truth is my identity' and refers to the practice of aligning with your internal power and truth as you awaken to your vital life force.

Ong - This word equates with the word creator and taps into the Kundalini, your primal creative life force.

Akal, Maha Kal - This mantra translates to mean, 'undying, great death,' which puts you into a relaxed state of mind and is also reinforces life force.

Sa Ta Na Ma -This mantra illustrates the five primal sounds of the whole of the Universe. Intoning this mantra will bring you into closer contact with all that is. Each letter related to a specific concept:

S = Infinity

T = Life

M = Rebirth

A = The 5TH sound is the first letter.

You can use all of these mantras throughout your Kundalini awakening practice. You can find more of these mantras as you expand your consciousness on all of the levels of Kundalini ascension.

Use mantras as often as needed to bring you into closer conscious alignment with divine source energy and your original true power.

Chapter 13 Energy Vortex

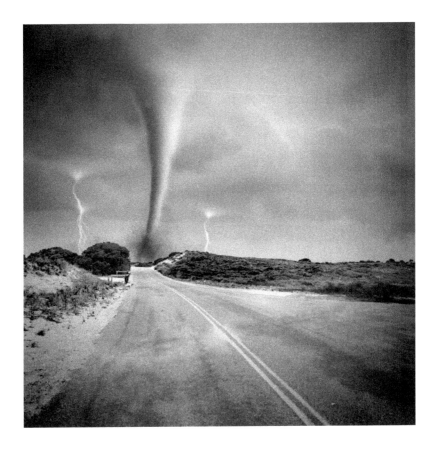

Everything on this planet radiates some energy, whether it is life force or not. These energies can often be seen radiating up to a foot off of whatever object from which they are originally attached. Seeing these energies is not tricky, but it does take practice. As long as we understand that these energies are all around us, we can use them to our advantage in meditation.

Many people might confuse the vibrational energies of chi with those of our Kundalini. Chi is essential in differentiating a corpse from a living being, acting more like the fire that ignites the flame of life within our bodies. Kundalini is more connected to the energies of our soul that interacts with our physical body. Even after death, we will take the unique energies and awakenings of our Kundalini with us. Chi will no longer exist in our physical being once we have passed on since the process would snuff out the flame of life.

Even though our chi is different from our Kundalini, it is necessary for our awakening. Without energy, there would be no power for our spirit to grow to awaken on a higher spiritual level. Understanding the power of all energies that fill our universe will help significantly in the advancement of our mental and spiritual growth. It is also said that if there is something wrong with or blocking our chi, it is a sign of ailment. To clear one's chi will help cure disease and cancers that harm our physical form so that we can feel extravagantly better.

Chi directly influences our Kundalini and, because of this, many techniques have been created to help improve the flow of our chi or life energy, improving the passage of vibrational energies that travel through our Nadi.

Tai Chi is the name of one of these very practices that help to improve the channel of our flame of life. Strengthening the core of our chi so that the fire inside of us can burn brighter and provide us with more energy. Tai Chi itself is a form of dance that helps us relax and visualize the flow of our energies. The ultimate balance of Yin and Yang is one of the main focuses of the practice of Tai Chi, making it extremely popular in the use of yoga regimes around the world.

To be able to practice the original teaching of Tai Chi, an individual will have to dedicate their time to memorizing one hundred and eight of the complicated moves. It has been proven that these types of practices help improve our physical balance and flexibility while also lowering both blood pressure and cholesterol.

Tai Chi has also been reported to help the enhancing of the release of serotonin and endorphins. This practice is very well known to have successful results in energizing individuals who use it. Strengthening our life force can only bring success to us while traveling down the path of spiritual awakening. Knowing how to use all of these different tools and practices available to us is vital to the excelling of our psychic abilities.

Depending on what type of meditation we choose to practice or what trials we are about to face, we can create our armory of helpful talismans and energies to help us through the process. The best way to harness these energies is through the natural elements of earth that Mother Nature gifts to us. Most rocks and crystals hold strong auras that can help enhance our abilities or even decrease the threat to others, but any creation of nature can help us in these ways.

It is always wise to keep grounding energy on or by us at all times, especially while meditating. Variants of these types of grounding energies are usually found from stones, plants, and animals. These beings of the earth will also help deflect any negativity that might try to find its way into our auric field.

For best results through this type of energy use, sticking to hard stones, crystals, and druses are always an ideal thing to do. Making sure that whichever stone we choose is within our line of vision in our meditational space is crucial as well, even if it is out of our peripheral vision. These rocks will help us feel physically and mentally better. Stones and crystals act as vessels for swells of energy, and these energies can be reflected both ways from human to stone.

If a stone ends up reflecting too much of us, it can become an unpleasant experience to use them for healing. This type of toxin is mainly caused by a type of "overload" in our crystals and can easily be fixed by a crystal cleanse. Stone and crystal cleansing and can be achieved through many various techniques, some of the most famous being to set the stones under the sun, or preferably the full or new moon, to recharge and clear the energies. There are many writings and teachings available that focus more on each rock and all the benefits they can bring to our spiritual growth.

The earth itself is completely built from vibrational energies that radiate from its very core. Being able to access these energies and powers is one of mother earth's many gifts of enlightenment and healing. We can always turn to the earth and its gift of life to help us shake loose the blockages that halt the current of our vibrational energies. Different rocks will give off very different vibrations that are all unique in their healing capabilities. It might be challenging to try to pin what energies we need to work with, but as long as we let the stones call out to our auric energies, we can never go wrong.

Many forms of literature exist to help list all of the stones and crystal available to man and all of their healing properties. Using these guides can help us narrow down exactly what areas in our energy that we want to focus on healing. It is also usually helpful to find stones that resonate with the color of the aura that we are trying to clear. For example, our sixth chakra, the heart chakra, is a deep green, so using green stones can help activate this energy and promote proper healing.

The rawer the stone, the more genuine and powerful the energies will be. Human hands, making them smoother and more aesthetically pleasing to the naked eye, tamper with a lot of stones and gems. This does not mean that the healing powers of the stone are removed, of course, but slightly muted so that their effects will not be as strong. There are many ways to "recharge" these stones, in a sense, using the powers of the earth, sun, and moon. Leaving stones in the rays of a full or new moon help considerably with charging their vibrational energies.

It is also a very wise idea to use dried white sage to smudge and clear any negativity within or around our stones. Keeping them near plants will also help heighten their vibrational energies, so having a small indoor garden would be ideal.

Using dried herbs and flowers are also hugely beneficial to the awakening and healing of our spiritual energies. Keeping a pouch of dried lavender at our side has been said to enhance one's ability to see spirits on the other side. Using lavender oils and flowers during our exercises will help ease anxiety and stress while also easing physical skin irritations.

Rosemary is also a beneficial plant as it acts as a sort of antiseptic. This plant can be used to help release our mental capabilities and help promote spiritual purification.

A more detailed list of crystals and their benefits are as follows:

- Amethyst – provides protection, spiritual purification, and spiritual well being.
- Blue tiger eye – Soothing, provides emotional balance, and clarity.
- Black obsidian – Promotes healing, protection, and grounding.
- Azurite – Promotes communication and intuition; provides guidance.
- Celestite – Helps with angelic communication, clarity, and our Devine   expression.
- Rhodochrosite – Provides comfort, compassion, and love.
- Bloodstone – Detoxifies physically and emotionally, promotes healing and grounding.
- Seraphinite (Serafina) – Helps us reach Divine ascension and connects us to the   Devic kingdom.
- Spirit (Cactus) Quartz – Creates a spiritual connection, unity, and harmony.
- Selenite – Promotes our Divine connection and our highest vibrations.
- Hematite – Extremely grounding and balancing; detoxifies body and mind.
- Picture Jasper – Inspires confidence and creative visualization.

- Sandstone – Helps promote creativity, mental and spiritual clarity, and unites us as a whole.
- Petrified wood – Provides strength and support, grounds energies.

A lot of these stones can be easily found in most jewelry and rock shops. The more positive vibrational energies will be within the stones that have been collected raw and haven't been processed or put through human made machines to "beautify" these stones give them a more glossed look. This is not to say that polished stones will not provide any vibrational healing energy, as every stone from Mother Earth will have the power and energy of Kundalini.

Kundalini herself is a form of vibrational energy. We can help wake her from her slumber by using different stones and crystals.

The best way to tell what kind of stone we need is to see which one we are most naturally drawn to while browsing in shops or natural areas. Our body's energies will reach out to those it needs, as long as we listen, we can find some handy tools for our meditation.

Stones in the form of jewelry are very helpful, as they will physically surround our aura with their different vibrations, which can provide protection against negativity as well as a boost for our aura.

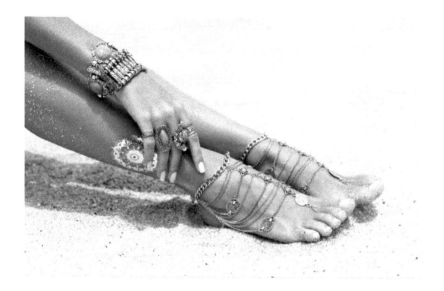

Creating a balanced meditation area will be extremely beneficial for the progress of our Kundalini Awakening, as long as it is a place that brings us calm and peace. Some people may prefer to be in the company of others by attending various Kundalini Yoga classes, and others achieve a much higher sense of awakening when they are secluded. While it is advised not to force ourselves into uncomfortable situations, it is always a good idea to test our limits and push the boundaries of our comfort zone even further. In doing so, we can learn new ways to help shake the closed gates of our spiritual channel.

If we do not have a particular place in mind for meditation, we can quickly create a peaceful environment on our own. For example, many people like to meditate in the warm waters of a bath or shower since it offers a lot of quiet and privacy, while also naturally relaxing the body.

Anywhere we choose to create our meditational environment; it is always a good idea to fill the area with various stones and crystals. Plants are also beneficial and cleansing to have present during our meditation. Not only do they visually bring calm to our mind, but they also can purify the air, which is extremely important for breathing exercises.

White sage is extraordinarily cleansing and will offer protection for embarking on our journey of awakening. Dried white sage can be used to smudge and cleanse the energies around and within our auric field. This cleansing power will help rid us of any harmful attachments and energies that might hinder our healing. Sometimes healing can make one feel extremely vulnerable as they face the trials of their awakening. Smudging and clearing our aura will help us keep a steadier mind and focus on healing our emotional, physical, and spiritual wounds.

A list of essential plants is as follows:

- Spider plant – air purification; removes carbon monoxide from the air.
- Rosemary – promotes happiness, improves memory, and combats fatigue.
- Fennel – courage, and strength.
- Chamomile – promotes healing.
- Marjoram – protection and happiness.
- Lavender – relieves anxiety and tension, slows heart rate, and alleviates headaches.
- Ivy – Cleanses air and relieves asthma.
- Basil – produces oxygen and absorbs toxins from the air.
- Oregano – stimulates healthy family relationships, happiness, and spiritual cleansing.

- Dracaena – Increases self-esteem, purifies the air, and focuses our physical and spiritual mind.
- Ficus – Represents unity and understanding; symbolizes peace.
- Jasmine – Triggers the heart chakra, boosts energies, improves productivity, and enhances one's self-esteem.
- Lily – cleanses physical, emotional, and spiritual problems; ideal for a bedroom environment as it stimulates tranquility.
- Sage – Promotes positive energy flow and cleanses negativity.
- Orchid – Brings positive energies to the home, spiritual wellbeing, provides oxygen, and romance.
- Money Plant – attracts wealth and good luck, alleviates stress; absorbs synthetic chemicals within the home.

These are only a few of the many plants that can help us on a spiritual level. If we have animals in our home, make sure that none of the plants that we gather are poisonous to them; Lilies are especially poisonous to cats. It is much safer to stick with the energies of herbs if we have animals that can reach them since those are almost always safe for our pets to consume.

It is also important to keep in mind the power of the essential oils extracted from the very plants themselves. We can use these oils to help draw the beneficial healing powers of the specific plant's essential oil that we choose to use. Many people will turn to the reliable Bach Flower Remedies as they are high-quality essential oils that offer strong vibrational powers. Mixing various plants and oils is also an excellent practice to make specific tinctures made from plants that will directly help us with the issue that we are facing. While some may not have complete faith in the healing power of oils, the proof will shine through in the form of improved health.

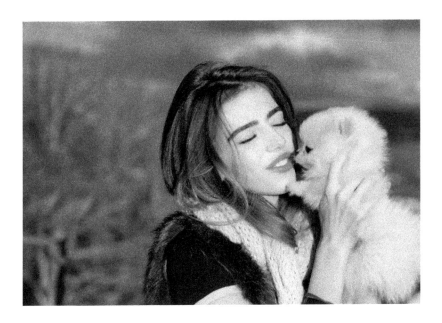

We have talked about the lavender plant as a sort of antianxiety and muscle relaxant, but it also has profound spiritual significance. Keeping a pouch of dried lavender on our person is said to enhance the ability of the third-eye and allow us to see and hear spirits more clearly.

As long as we understand the powers of the earth and the effects it can have on human beings, we can take advantage of the vibrational healing properties. Even certain animals can help guide us through our lessons of awakening.

There are many guides available to us as long as we are open to receiving their wisdom. If there is an animal that keeps showing up in our life, whether physically or in a photo or name, we can research what messages this particular being is trying to teach us.

For a straightforward example, signs of crickets, frogs, and toads can represent leaps forward within our life and spiritual healing. Frogs and toads also give us the lesson of metamorphosis and change in our lives. There are many forms of literature available to us that focus on the energies and lessons of the animals and insects that present themselves to us. Messages from the creatures of the earth are indeed precious gifts and should be treated as such.

Conclusion

The right time is now. Pick something you have learned in the book and start working on it. Remember, you have to continuously practice in order to succeed, so you have to schedule the time to do so.

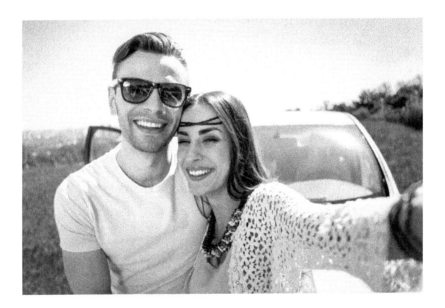

You cannot rush the process. Take it slow and enjoy how things go. Try to learn as much as you possibly can from this process. Chances are, you are going to learn things about yourself that you were not previously aware of. Use this book as a guide for your journey to awakening.

No two people's journey is going to be the same, so make it your own. Go where your higher self tells you to go. Even the simplest meditation exercise can be practiced for decades without losing its potency and power.

This shows the immense amount of potential that humans have to transform their lives and empower themselves that these practices have to offer.

Take care to be selfless and grateful for these practices, as they have found you for a distinct reason. And always remember to stay in the present moment, "Wherever you are, you live fully in the here and now."

That this book can help you to improve your life.

CPSIA information can be obtained
at www.ICGtesting.com
Printed in the USA
LVHW051728080221
678722LV00013B/2106